T0239384

Cochlear Implantation for Common Cavity Deformity

Yongxin Li
Editor

Cochlear Implantation for Common Cavity Deformity

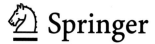 Springer

Editor
Yongxin Li
Department of Otorhinolaryngology Head and Neck Surgery
Beijing Tongren Hospital
Capital Medical University
Beijing, China

ISBN 978-981-16-8219-3   ISBN 978-981-16-8217-9   (eBook)
https://doi.org/10.1007/978-981-16-8217-9

This Springer imprint is published by the registered company Springer Nature Singapore Pte Ltd.
The registered company address is: 152 Beach Road, #21-01/04 Gateway East, Singapore 189721,
Singapore

Foreword

Cochlear implant is one of the most famous bionic products in the twentieth century. China's first cochlear implantation was carried out in 1995. At present, there are more than 800,000 cochlear implant users in the world, and near 90,000 cases in China. The development of cochlear implantation technology is an important event that is able to be beneficial to the national economy and people's livelihood and it can improve the comprehensive quality of the population.

Inner ear malformation is a complicated problem in cochlear implantation. The author of this book, Professor Yongxin Li from Cochlear Implant Center of Beijing Tongren Hospital, has been devoted to the clinical and technical research of difficult cochlear implantation for many years, especially in case of severe inner ear malformations, such as common cavity deformity and cochlear nerve deficiency, and has made some new achievements. He is recognized as the first one in China to use the transmastoid labyrinthotomy approach with customized electrodes for common cavity deformity. After long-term follow-up, the author found the patients with common cavity deformity achieved good postoperative results by combining the surgical approach and special electrode. After the author's promotion, now his method has applied in many places in China and will benefit more such kind of patients.

The book *Cochlear Implantation for Common Cavity Deformity* introduces the basic discovery and related clinical practice of common cavity deformity in detail, and systematically discusses the development, perioperative evaluation, surgical strategies, and postoperative outcomes of cochlear implantation technology. What's more, the author presents the experience of auditory assessment and postoperative follow-up results in this kind of patients from Beijing Tongren Hospital, which makes the book more valuable and offer new insights for clinical application.

Zhengmin Wang
Professor,
Department of Otolaryngology,
Eye and ENT Hospital of Fudan University,
Shanghai, China

Foreword

In 1972, the world's first generation of single-channel cochlear implant was born, bringing hope for patients with severe deafness to regain hearing. Ten years later, the multichannel cochlear implant that truly restored hearing to the deaf was approved by the FDA and became the most representative biomedical engineering device to date.

Around the world, nearly 900,000 people have received cochlear implants, more than half of them were children. In China, up to 90% of cochlear implants users were children. Beijing Tongren Hospital is a large-scale cochlear implantation and technical training center. Since the successful implantation of the first child cochlear implant users in China in 1997, cochlear implant has been successfully performed on more than 5,000 deafness patients in our center, among which up to 45% are patients with inner ear malformations, thus we have rich experience for inner ear malformation implantation.

Professor Yongxin Li, author of *Cochlear implantation for Common Cavity Deformity*, was the earliest participant of the Cochlear Implant Center at Beijing Tongren Hospital and the doctor who has performed the most cochlear implants. For more than 20 years, he has been specializing in cochlear implant technology and has participated in many technical training and academic exchanges around the world and accumulated rich clinical experience. Due to the special academic influence of our hospital, nearly half of the deaf patients waiting for cochlear implantation were accompanied with inner ear malformations, including severe malformation, such as common cavity deformity. Severe anatomical variation of common cavity deformity makes it difficult to implant electrodes easily, and it is easy to cause facial nerve injury and cerebrospinal fluid otorrhea, which makes cochlear implantation for common cavity being a technical highland. Therefore, Professor Yongxin Li led his team to research and solve the key problems and he was the first in China to implant customized electrodes through transmastoid labyrinthotomy approach, which shortened the operation time, controlled surgical complications, and achieved satisfactory treatment results.

Cochlear implantation for Common cavity deformity, a book with technical features, includes a detailed introduction of cochlear implantation for common cavity deformity. The author focused on the embryo development, pre- and postoperative audiology and radiology evaluation, surgical method, electrode design, postoperative auditory ability, and vestibular function evaluation of common cavity deformity. At the same time, it also vividly introduces the preoperative auditory training and evaluation methods and postoperative programming strategies of such patients.

We hope that the publication of this new book will provide more technical reference for otologist and help them to successfully carry out cochlear implantation surgery for patients with common cavity malformation.

Demin Han
Department of Otorhinolaryngology Head and Neck Surgery,
Beijing Tongren Hospital, Capital Medical University,
Beijing, China

Key Laboratory of Otolaryngology Head and Neck Surgery
(Capital Medical University), Ministry of Education,
Beijing, China

Preface

Cochlear implantation (CI) with inner ear malformations has always been the difficulty of cochlear implantation, and common cavity deformity (CCD) is one of the most severe inner ear malformations. Previous experience has found that CI for CCD has high difficulty and poor postoperative results. Beijing Tongren Hospital, as one of the cochlear implant centers that carry out CI surgery at the earliest and perform the largest number of operations in China, has received more and more difficult CI patients in recent years, which has increased from 17% to 60% in recent years. In difficult CI, inner ear malformation accounts for 90%. Therefore, the quantity and quality of patients with CCD are among the best in the world. Due to urgent clinical needs, after many years of clinical research and accumulation, and communication with related scholars all around the world, I used the most suitable operation approach and accompanied with customized electrode for CCD patients and achieved good outcomes. At present, our center has more than 50 cases of CCD patients implanted CI, and has carried on regular follow-up for many years, some results will be presented in this book.

Due to the special anatomical structure of CCD and often accompanied with cochlear nerve deficiency, its surgical strategy, postoperative programming, postoperative outcome, and pre- and postoperative vestibular and balance functions are all special. Therefore, this book will comprehensively introduce the CCD from the aspects of embryo development, preoperative audiological assessment and auditory training, radiology research progress, surgical technique development, postoperative programming strategy, postoperative outcome research progress, and postoperative vestibular and balance function. Combined with specific cases, the specific surgical methods, postoperative programming, and auditory and speech development will be introduced. The book provides a lot of surgery and programming pictures, vividly showing the relevant experience of the center.

Although CCD for a small proportion of inner ear malformations, its treatment principles and experience can be extended to patients with cochlear nerve deficiency and other inner ear malformations, and the mastery of CCD by all surgeons can benefit more patients. In addition, it is our great honor to invite Academicians Zhengmin Wang and Demin Han to check and preface this book. Academician Zhengmin Wang is one of the first scholars in the research of CI technology and equipment in China. He has been devoted to the research of domestic cochlear implant for many years and has made considerable achievements. He has rich experience in CI surgery and is the one of the most outstanding audiologists among the older generation. Academician Demin Han is the first academician of Beijing Tongren Hospital, and he led the Otolaryngology Department achieving a number of technical breakthroughs; the first domestic children CI surgery was completed in our hospital under his guidance. After that, the CI surgery technology of our hospital progressed gradually, and the related research also developed steadily, until today, we made many achievements. We hope the book *Cochlear Implantation for Common Cavity Deformity* can provide useful reference for otologists all around the world. If you have any comments, please contact me. Thank you.

Beijing, China   Yongxin Li

Contents

Embryology of Inner Ear Malformation Types and its Radiological Relevance

Anandhan Dhanasingh

1.1 Introduction

Embryology is the basis for understanding the intimate relation between anatomical structures in different organ systems and is the basis for understanding disorders of development. Inner ear starts to form at the beginning of 3rd week and develops further with the two-and-half turns of the cochlear duct and three semicircular canals of the vestibular organ at the end of 8th week of embryogenesis (Jackler et al. 1987). Inner ear malformation of various degrees depends on the time of arrest in the differentiation or development of inner ear structures (Bartel-Friedrich et al. 2007). Understanding the embryology of the inner ear would help to identify the stage of development/differentiation arrest, a malformed inner ear has encountered. This will further support the decision-making of treating with cochlear implants or not. This chapter will start by describing the embryologic development of the human inner ear in brief based on earlier literature. The later part of this chapter will focus mainly on the embryology of all the malformation types including the common cavity malformation with several example cases with variable degrees of structural development.

1.2 Embryology of Inner Ear

Inner ear starts to form between 3rd and 4th week of gestation which is much earlier than the external ear development that starts at the 7th week of gestation (Jackler et al. 1987). The first sign of inner ear development happens around the end of the 3rd

The original version of this chapter was revised. The correction to this chapter can be found at https://doi.org/10.1007/978-981-16-8217-9_11

A. Dhanasingh (✉)
MED-EL Medical Electronics GmbH, Innsbruck, Austria
e-mail: Anandhan.Dhanasingh@medel.com

week, by a thickening of the outside layer of ectoderm, on each side of the cephalic end. This grouping of cells in the auditory placode or otic placode and is genetically programmed to become the membranous labyrinth at a later stage. As programmed, the placode invaginates inward to form the auditory pit or otic pit. The otic pit invaginates further and gets completely encircled in mesoderm and forms the otocyst by the end of 4th week. Figure 1.1a shows the formation of otic placode, otic pit, and otocyst. The ventral portion of the otocyst gives rise to the saccule and the cochlear duct, and the dorsal portion of the otocyst forms the utricle and semicircular canals (SCC), and endolymphatic duct. During the 5th week, the lower pole of the saccule starts to lengthen and coil. This projection, the cochlear duct, penetrates the surrounding mesenchyme in a spiral fashion. In the 6th week, the semicircular canals begin as folded evaginations of membrane from the dorsal side of the otocyst. The superior SCC (SSCC) is the first to form, followed by the posterior and then lateral canal. By the end of 6th week, the vestibular portion develops further giving rise to the three distinct semicircular canals of the vestibular organ. The cochlear portion as well starts to elongate at this time point. By the end of 8th week, the cochlear duct has made two-and-half turns along with the cochlear aqueduct.

During the 7th week, cochlear duct epithelial cells differentiate to form the Organ of Corti. These epithelial cells are initially similar, but with time, they differentiate into inner and outer ridges. The inner ridge becomes the future osseous spiral lamina and the outer ridge goes on to develop the inner and outer hair cells. The stereocilia of the hair cells are contacted by the tectorial membrane, which attaches to the spiral lamina. The spiral ganglion cells also differentiate from cells in the wall of cochlear duct, which migrate along the coiled membranous cochlea to form the

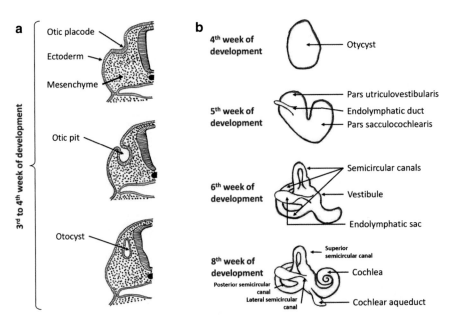

Fig. 1.1 The inner ear starts its formation at the beginning of 3rd week developing the otic placode which invaginates forming the otocyst by the end of 4th week (**a**). The otocyst further differentiates/develops and reaches two-and-half turns of the cochlear duct and three distinct semicircular canals of the vestibular portion by the end of 8th week of gestation (**b**)

ganglion. Mesenchyme surrounding the cochlear duct soon differentiates into cartilage. During the 10th week, this cartilaginous tissue undergoes vacuolization and forms the two perilymphatic spaces: the scala vestibuli and scala tympani (Oliver and Kesser 2013). Meanwhile, the labyrinth continues to expand rapidly, so that near the end of the 5th month, the inner ear is close to adult size. Thus, the cochlea grows to its full size in a span of six months (Peck 1994).

The development of the cochlear-vestibular nerve and of the central auditory system is less understood. Ganglion cells from the auditory nerve (8th nerve) emerge from the otocyst in the 4th week of gestation. These fibers start to enter the expanding cochlea in the 5th week. This is followed by the cochlear branch of the auditory nerve fans out in parallel to the curving cochlea. Peripheral dendrites in the basal portion of the cochlea start to get connected with inner hair cells between 11th and 12th week. Whereas, at the cochlear apex, the spiral fibers contact the base of the outer hair cells in 14th week. All synapses are formed by the 7th month of pregnancy, and maturation of contact between cochlea and peripheral nerves takes place in the last trimester. The sensorineural system is matured enough to permit experiencing the sensation of sound between the 6th and the 7th month. The internal auditory canal (IAC) is formed by inhibition of cartilage formation at the medial aspect of the otic vesicle. This inhibition requires the presence of the vestibulocochlear nerve. In the absence of the eighth nerve, IAC will not be formed (Peck 1994; Amarnath et al. 2016).

1.3   Inner Ear Malformation Types and Time of Developmental Arrest

Inner ear malformation types are the result of developmental arrest at various time points of the embryology (Bartel-Friedrich et al. 2007). This section will discuss the time of developmental arrest associated with key inner ear malformation types that are well reported in the literature.

Michel's deformity or also called complete labyrinthine aplasia refers to the absence of entire inner ear structures including the internal auditory canal (IAC) (Fig. 1.2). Such a severe malformation type is very rare and is thought to occur due

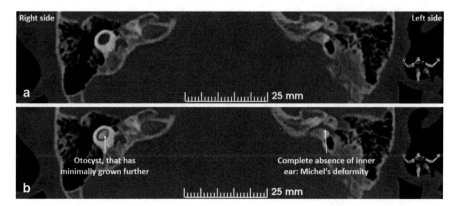

Fig. 1.2 Axial view of the temporal bone showing a rudimentary otocyst on the right-side ear and complete absence of the inner ear structures on the left-side ear. Computer tomography (CT) image slice (**a**) and three-dimensional (3D) segmented image of the inner ear (**b**)

to the developmental arrest of otic placode early in the 3rd week of gestation (Yiin et al. 2011). Figure 1.2 shows the right-side ear with a rudimentary otocyst and left-side ear with a complete absence of inner ear structures. Cochlear implantation (CI) is contraindicated in this type of malformation, and auditory brainstem implantation (ABI) may be considered as an option.

Cochlear aplasia (CA) refers to the complete absence of the cochlear portion with a normal or malformed vestibular portion and IAC. The arrest of otic placode, late in the 3rd week of gestation results in CA. This is how it is reported in majority of the literature (Amarnath et al. 2016; Yiin et al. 2011; Mazón et al. 2017). But we think that the otic placode develops further into the otocyst. At this stage, the ventral portion of the otocyst stops developing further resulting in the absence of the cochlear portion. Whereas the dorsal portion of the otocyst develops further forming the vestibular organ at the end of the 6th week. If the vestibular portion is normally developed with three distinct semicircular canals, then it is contraindicated for placing the CI electrode inside the vestibular organ. ABI may be considered as an option (Fig. 1.3).

In case if the vestibular portion appears as a single cavity, this may allow the CI electrode to be safely inserted, making a nice loop with the stimulating contacts placed close to the wall of the cavity as shown in Fig. 1.4 (*left side*), where the neural elements are believed to be present (Graham et al. 2000). The vestibular cavity with no clear distinction in the formation of three semicircular canals is the result of developmental arrest during the 6th week of gestation. Often in the CI field, the vestibular cavity as shown in Fig. 1.4 is misunderstood as a common cavity malformation (Weiss et al. 2021).

In some cases, the developmental arrest of the inner ear structures is seen only on one side, with normal development of inner ear on the other side. Figure 1.5 is an

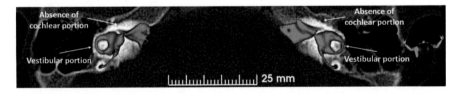

Fig. 1.3 Axial view of temporal bone showing the absence of the cochlear portion (CA) and the presence of vestibular organ with three distinct semicircular canals

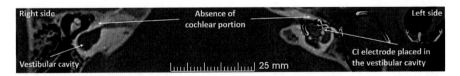

Fig. 1.4 Axial view of the temporal bone showing the absence of the cochlear portion (CA) but the presence of a vestibular organ in the form of a cavity. The left side ear shows the electrode placement in the form of a loop inside the vestibular cavity

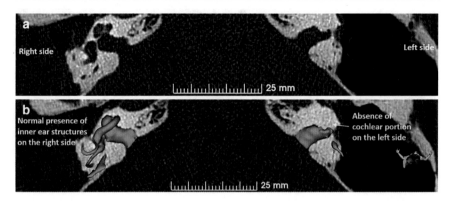

Fig. 1.5 Axial view of the temporal bone showing normal presence of the inner ear on the right side and cochlear aplasia on the left side. CT image slice (**a**) and 3D segmented image of the inner ear (**b**)

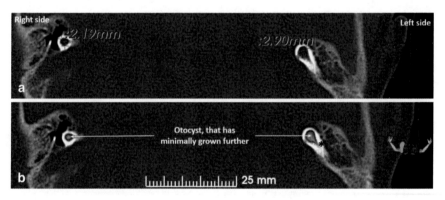

Fig. 1.6 Otocyst on both sides with no further development as seen from the axial view of CT image slice (**a**) and 3D segmented image (**b**)

example case showing a normal presence of inner ear on the right side and CA on the left side.

Common cavity (CC) malformation is due to the developmental arrest of otocyst during the 4th week of gestation. Though there is no differentiation between the cochlea and the vestibule at this stage, both together forming a large cystic cavity with no internal architecture, but there will be overall growth in the size of the cavity. There could be some developments in the SCCs during the 6th week. Figure 1.6 shows a case with a developmental arrest right at the 4th week with a very minimal further growth in the overall size of the cavity. The dorsal end of the otocyst on the left side, however, shows a glimpse of development into vestibular portion but failed in its attempt. Such a small-sized cavity will contraindicate CI as the cavity size is too small to accommodate any electrode.

Figure 1.7 shows bilateral CC grown to its full size with the presence of posterior SCC on the right side and lateral SCC on the left side. The cavity is fluid filled with

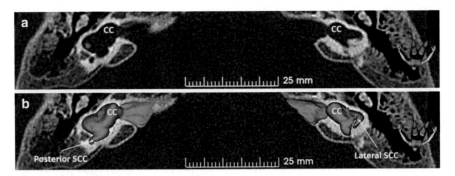

Fig. 1.7 Axial view of the temporal bone showing bilateral CC malformation. Posterior SCC on the right-side ear and lateral SCC on the left-side ear are seen additionally developed. CT image slice (**a**) and 3D segmented image of the inner ear (**b**)

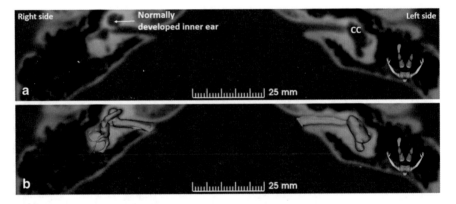

Fig. 1.8 Axial view of the temporal bone showing normally developed inner ear on the right ear and developmental arrest of otocyst at the end of 4th week leaving a CC malformation on the left side. CT image slice (**a**) and 3D segmented image of the inner ear (**b**)

no clear understanding on the presence of sensorineural elements. However, the literature reports on the presence of neural elements along the wall of the cavity (Graham et al. 2000) and therefore a CI electrode is proposed to be placed close to the wall of the cavity as shown in Fig. 1.4. A pre-curved electrode with the contacts facing the inner curvature of the electrode may not be effective at least theoretically.

Figure 1.8 is an example showing the developmental arrest of otocyst at the end of 4th week of gestation leaving a CC malformation on the left side and normally developed inner ear on the right side.

Incomplete Partition type I (IP type I) malformation or otherwise called as cystic cochleovestibular malformation is the result of the developmental arrest of otocyst in 5th week (Mazón et al. 2017). The otocyst starts to divide during the 5th week into cochlear and vestibular portions separately but the developmental arrest prevents further development. This separation of cochlear and vestibular portion in

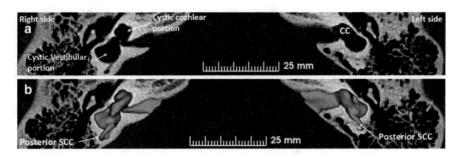

Fig. 1.9 Axial view of the temporal bone showing IP type I malformation on the right-side ear and CC malformation on the left-side ear. IP type I on the right side shows a cystic cochlear portion and dilated vestibular portion. CT image slice (**a**) and 3D segmented image of the inner ear (**b**)

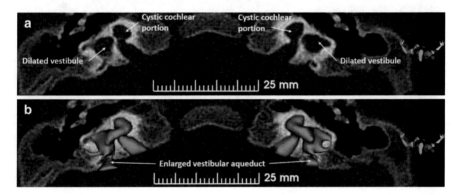

Fig. 1.10 Axial view of the temporal bone with bilateral IP type I malformation showing cystic cochlear portion and dilated vestibule. CT image slice (**a**) and 3D segmented image of the inner ear showing enlarged vestibular aqueduct (**b**)

IP type I distinguishes it from CC malformation. The cochlear portion lacks the entire modiolus giving a cystic appearance as shown in Fig. 1.9, right side ear. Figure 1.9 shows the CC malformation type on the left side which is the result of developmental arrest of otocyst by the end of 4th week of gestation with no further development of the inner ear. There is no clear understanding on the presence of sensorineural elements inside the cystic cochlea. Scientific reports on the hearing performance of IP type-I malformation patients with CI, give the hope that there are neural elements probably along the wall of the cystic cochlea that are potent enough to capture the electrical stimulation from the CI electrode (Eftekharian et al. 2019).

Figure 1.10 is another example of IP type I malformation bilaterally showing dilated vestibular aqueduct (VA). Dilated VA is the result of developmental arrest between 5th and 6th weeks of gestation. The 5th and 6th week of gestation plays a role in the formation of IP type I malformation and the enlarged VA.

Cochlear Hypoplasia (CH) is the result of developmental arrest in the 6th week of gestation and is configured by the differentiation of semicircular canals of vestibular portion and the elongation of cochlear duct. Figure 1.11a refers to a

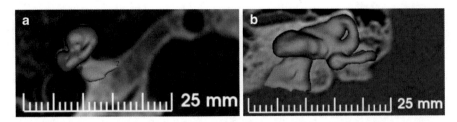

Fig. 1.11 Axial view of the hypoplastic cochlea. Vestibular portion is completely absent, and the basal turn of the cochlear portion is developed (**a**). The vestibular portion is normally developed with minimal development in the cochlear portion (**b**)

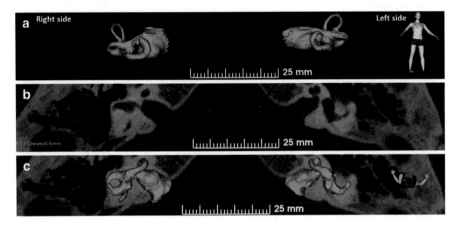

Fig. 1.12 CT image slice in the axial view (**a**). The 3D segmented image of the inner ear is shown in the axial plane (**b**) and the coronal plane (**c**)

mushroom-shaped cochlear portion with a clear absence of the vestibular portion. This can be explained by the developmental arrest of the dorsal portion of the otocyst between 5th and 6th week of gestation stopping the vestibular portion to develop whereas the ventral portion of the otocyst developed further forming the basal portion of the cochlea. Figure 1.11b shows the hypoplastic cochlea with almost normal development of the vestibular portion and minimally developed cochlear portion. This can be explained by the developmental arrest of the ventral portion of the otocyst in the 6th week preventing the cochlear duct to further elongate, whereas the dorsal portion of the otocyst developed further to form the three distinct SCCs of the vestibular portion.

Figure 1.12 is another example of cochlear hypoplasia type malformation with almost normal presence of vestibular portion bilaterally, but the cochlear portion encountered developmental arrest at different time points. The right-side cochlea is developed for less than one full turn whereas the left-side cochlea is seen developed up to one-and-half turns as shown in Fig. 1.12a in the coronal view. This can be explained assuming the development arrest earlier in the 6th week on the right side and later in the 6th week on the left side. Figure 1.12b and c shows the axial view of the inner ear as seen in both in CT image slice and in 3D segmentation, respectively.

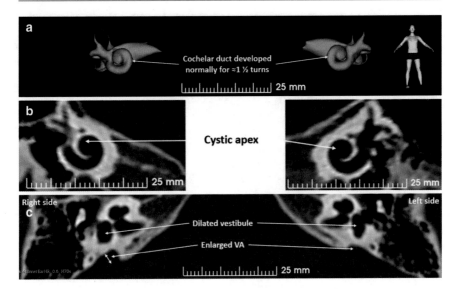

Fig. 1.13 3D segmented inner ear in the coronal plane showing the cochlear duct developed normally for the basal 1 ½ turns (**a**). The CT image slice in the coronal plane shows the cystic apex (**b**). CT image slice in the axial view showing dilated vestibule and enlarged VA (**c**)

The cochlear duct epithelial cells are expected to differentiate and form the sensorineural elements starting from the 7th week of gestation inside the cochlear portion, which is developed to various degrees (Sennaroglu 2016) as shown in Figs. 1.11 and 1.12. If the cochlear nerve presence is confirmed from the sagittal view of the magnetic resonance imaging (MRI), then the CI is expected to offer hearing benefits to the recipients.

Incomplete Partition type II (IP type II) or otherwise called as Mondini's deformation is due to the developmental arrest of otocyst during 7th week of gestation. Until 7th week, the cochlear duct grows to almost one-and-half turns as shown in Fig. 1.13a. At this point, the developmental arrest happens to stop further growth and as a result, the middle and the apical portion of the cochlea appears as a cystic apex as shown in Fig. 1.13b. In most cases, the vestibular portion is fully formed although the vestibule is dilated, and the VA is seen enlarged in majority of the IP type II cases as shown in Fig. 1.13c. The enlarged VA (>1.5 mm measured at the midpoint of external aperture) is explained by the developmental arrest of endolymphatic duct during fifth and sixth week of gestation stopping the VA to get narrower.

The enlarged VA could lead to endolymphatic oozing during the CI electrode insertion as it has been reported (Vassoler et al. 2008). An electrode array length of 20 mm or 24 mm matching the 1 or 1 ½ turns of the cochlea would be a safe choice as inserting further into the cystic apex could end up with electrode tip fold-over as reported (Alsughayer et al. 2020).

Incomplete Partition type III (IP type III) or otherwise called as X-linked malformation is a genetically inherited disease linked to chromosome X and it is not

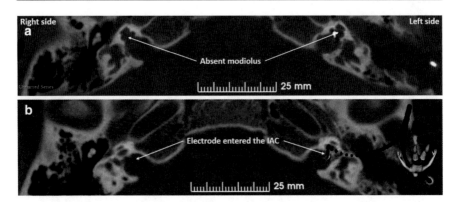

Fig. 1.14 Axial view of the temporal bone with IP type III malformation showing the complete absence of the central modiolus trunk (**a**). The tip of the CI electrode is seen inside the IAC on the left side (**b**)

due to the developmental arrest of the otocyst. The cochlea has inter-scalar septa but with a complete absence of the central modiolus trunk creating an open channel between the cochlea and the IAC (Corvino et al. 2018) as shown in Fig. 1.14a. Also, the IAC is seen enlarged. As a result, the chances are high for the cerebrospinal fluid gusher and CI electrode to enter the IAC as shown in Fig. 1.14b. It is unclear on the intracochlear organization of spiral ganglion neurons and other neural tissues but hearing performance with CI indicates the presence of sensorineural elements (Smeds et al. 2017).

1.4   Conclusion

The inner ear starts developing from the 3rd week and by the 8th week of gestation, the cochlear duct makes the two-and-half turns. Various degrees of inner ear malformation are the result of otic placode/otocyst developmental arrest at different time points in the embryology of inner ear. The common cavity, the most severe malformation type that is possible to treat with CI, is the result of developmental arrest in the 4th week. Whereas the mildest form of malformation type which is IP type II is the result of developmental arrest in the 7th week of gestation. IP type I and cochlear hypoplasia are the result of developmental arrest in the 5th and 6th week of gestation, respectively.

References

Alsughayer L, Al-Shawi Y, Yousef M, Hagr A. Cochlear electrode array tip fold-over in incomplete partition-I—A case report. Int J Pediatr Otorhinolaryngol. 2020 Dec;139:110438.
Amarnath C, Sathyan G, Soniya R, Periakaruppan AL, Shankar KS. Evaluation of embryological sequences of ear anomalies and its radiological relevance. Indian J Otol. 2016;22:248–57.

Bartel-Friedrich S, Wulke C. Classification and diagnosis of ear malformations. GMS Curr Top Otorhinolaryngol Head Neck Surg. 2007;6: Doc05. Epub 2008 Mar 14. PMID: 22073081; PMCID: PMC3199848.

Corvino V, Apisa P, Malesci R, Laria C, Auletta G, Franzé A. X-linked sensorineural hearing loss: a literature review. Curr Genomics. 2018 Aug;19(5):327–38.

Eftekharian A, Eftekharian K, Mokari N, Fazel M. Cochlear implantation in incomplete partition type I. Eur Arch Otorhinolaryngol. 2019 Oct;276(10):2763–8.

Graham JM, Phelps PD, Michaels L. Congenital malformations of the ear and cochlear implantation in children: review and temporal bone report of common cavity. J Laryngol Otol Suppl. 2000;25:1–14.

Jackler RK, Luxford WM, House WF. Congenital malformations of the inner ear: a classification based on embryogenesis. Laryngoscope. 1987 Mar;97(3 Pt 2 Suppl 40):2–14.

Mazón M, Pont E, Montoya-Filardi A, Carreres-Polo J, Más-Estellés F. Inner ear malformations: a practical diagnostic approach. Radiologia. 2017 Jul–Aug;59(4):297–305.

Oliver ER, Kesser BW. Embryology of ear (general). In: Kountakis SE, editor. Encyclopedia of otolaryngology, head and neck surgery. Berlin, Heidelberg: Springer; 2013.

Peck JE. Development of hearing. Part II. Embryology. J Am Acad Audiol. 1994;5:359–65.

Sennaroglu L. Histopathology of inner ear malformations: do we have enough evidence to explain pathophysiology? Cochlear Implants Int. 2016;17(1):3–20.

Smeds H, Wales J, Asp F, Löfkvist U, Falahat B, Anderlid BM, Anmyr L, Karltorp E. X-linked malformation and Cochlear implantation. Otol Neurotol. 2017 Jan;38(1):38–46.

Vassoler TM, Bergonse Gda F, Meira Junior S, Bevilacqua MC, Costa Filho OA. Cochlear implant and large vestibular aqueduct syndrome in children. Braz J Otorhinolaryngol. 2008 Mar–Apr;74(2):260–4.

Weiss NM, Langner S, Mlynski R, Roland P, Dhanasingh A. Evaluating common cavity Cochlear deformities using CT images and 3D reconstruction. Laryngoscope. 2021 Feb;131(2):386–91.

Yiin RS, Tang PH, Tan TY. Review of congenital inner ear abnormalities on CT temporal bone. Br J Radiol. 2011;84:859–63.

Preoperative Audiological Evaluation and Auditory Training for Patients with Common Cavity Deformity

2

Xingmei Wei, Haizhen Li, Shujin Xue, Jingyuan Chen, Yongxin Li, Ying Kong, and Sha Liu

Before cochlear implantation (CI), audiological assessment and radiology evaluation are necessary, because the condition of cochlear anatomy and auditory nerve need to be clarified. In this chapter, we introduce objective and subjective hearing assessment methods and results for common cavity deformity (CCD), and further describe if there were no residual hearing observed, the routine and characteristic means in our center.

2.1 Assessment of Objective Hearing

The objective hearing assessments methods are listed as follows:

- Acoustic immittance measurement: including tympanum curve and acoustic reflex threshold.

X. Wei (✉) · S. Xue · J. Chen · Y. Li
Department of Otorhinolaryngology Head and Neck Surgery, Beijing Tongren Hospital, Capital Medical University, Beijing, China

Key Laboratory of Otolaryngology Head and Neck Surgery (Capital Medical University), Ministry of Education, Beijing, China

H. Li
Department of pediatrics, Beijing Tongren Hospital, Capital Medical University, Beijing, China

Y. Kong · S. Liu
Key Laboratory of Otolaryngology Head and Neck Surgery (Capital Medical University), Ministry of Education, Beijing, China

Beijing Institute of Otolaryngology, Beijing Tongren Hospital, Capital Medical University, Beijing, China

- Auditory brainstem response (ABR). If possible, perform frequency-specific ABR.
- Distorted product otoacoustic emission (DPOAE). DPOAE can reflect the function of outer hair cells of the cochlea, but it can be affected by the condition of middle ear and external auditory canal.
- Cochlear microphonic (CM). CM can reflect the function of outer hair cells of the cochlea regardless of the condition of the middle ear. CM and OPOAE together can reflect the function of cochlear hair cells.
- 40 Hz auditory evoked related potential (40 Hz AERP).
- Multiple-frequency auditory steady-state responses (ASSR). For patients under 18 years old, if the frequency-specific ABR is not tested, the ASSR is needed to reflect the objective hearing levels for different frequencies.

All tests were carried out in a sound insulation room with background noise $\leq$30 dB (A). For children who cannot cooperate, 10% chloral hydrate (0.5 grams per kilogram of body weight) is given orally or enema for the objective hearing assessment, and the examinations were carried out when the children were sleeping.

Previous studies have shown that many patients with CCD have no meaningful objective residual hearing before surgery, and acoustic reflex, DPOAE, and 40 Hz AERP were all absent and ABR and ASSR were absent or present at 120 dB nHL (Xia et al. 2015). In our center, we count 51 CCD patients' objective hearing tests and the results are listed in Table 2.1. The results showed that less than 20% of patients had residual hearing. In ASSR test, 9 were positive in 500 Hz, 10 were positive in 1 k Hz, 7 were positive in 2 k Hz, 4 were positive in 4 k Hz; for 40 Hz AERP, 5 patients can elicit residual hearing; for ABR, 2 patients' residual hearing can be elicited. All the results showed that the objective residual hearing of CCD patients is usually poor.

2.2   Assessment of Subjective Hearing

For patients over 6 years who can cooperate with pure tone audiometry (PTA), PTAs were performed. For patients under 6 years, behavioral hearing assessments are performed, which include behavior observation audiometry (BOA), visual reinforcement audiometry (VRA), and play audiometry (PA). Both naked and aided subjective hearing tests shoulde be performed. Some works of literature have shown

Table 2.1   The objective hearing tests results of 51 CCD patients

	ASSR (Hz)				40 Hz AERP	AC ABR	BC ABR	CM	DPOAE
	500	1000	2000	4000					
N(P/T)	9/51	10/51	7/51	4/51	5/51	1/51	1/51	0/51	0/51
Percentage (%)	17.6	19.6	13.7	7.8	9.8	2.0	2.0	0	0

N = number, P = positive, T = total, ASSR = Multiple-frequency auditory steady-state responses, 40 Hz AERP = 40 Hz auditory evoked related potential, AC = air conductive, BC = bone conductive, ABR = Auditory brainstem response, DPOAE = Distorted product otoacoustic emission that the average PTA thresholds of CCD patients were ≥ 100 dB HL (Xia et al. 2015; Wei et al. 2018; Shi et al. 2019). We have collected 19 CCD patients' PTA results, and 8 can elicit subjective hearing, but the average hearing threshold was 105 dB HL, which may be caused by vibration.

2.3 Electrically Evoked Auditory Brainstem Responses

If a patient with CND has no response to objective or subjective hearing tests, electrically evoked auditory brainstem responses (EABR) can be used to determine whether their auditory pathway is integrity. EABR is generated by electricity and homologous to ABR anatomically and electrophysiologically. The slopes and peak amplitude correlated with neuronal survival (Mason et al. 1997). In clinical, for a special case like CCD, if there were good EABR waves, the peripheral auditory pathway was complete and CI was feasible. However, in some cases, no preoperative EABR eliciting can benefit from CI (Nikolopoulos et al. 2000), which indicated failure to elicit EABR is not a CI contraindication. This may be because EABR is easily interfered by the test environment. In addition, EABR test is usually done under anesthesia, and the stimulating electrode is placed in promontory, so the test is invasive. All above limit EABR's apply.

2.4 Preoperative Auditory Training

To overcome the defect of EABR, from 2003, our center proposed preoperative auditory training for CND patients with no preoperative residual hearing. Because CCD patients are often accompanied by CND, if the patient cannot be detected residual hearing, a high-power hearing aid can be worn for training. The hearing aid is selected by a professional audiologist and usually needs to be worn on both ears. A professional pediatrician and audiologist will train and observe the patient for 3 to 6 months to determine that the patient can respond to sounds. Only if they can respond to acoustic stimulation with a hearing aid, we can do CI surgery. At initial, the training period usually lasted for at least three months, now with social development and successful experience of CI surgery for CND, we could do CI surgery once the patients performed response to hearing. Usually for most CCD patients, after training they can get auditory response. If after training, the patient still has no hearing, preoperative EABR can be a choice to determine CI or auditory brainstem implant (ABI). But before birth of non-tumor ABI, to prolong training period was an alternate choice. As far as we know, the first approved ABI in China was performed in February 2019.

To sum up the above, the strategy of CI determination for CCD patients in our center is shown in Fig. 2.1.

Next, methods and outcomes of auditory training will be introduced.

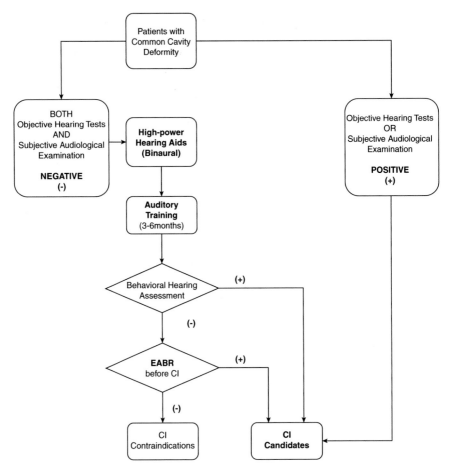

Fig. 2.1 The audiological assessment flow diagram of common cavity deformity for cochlear implantation determination

2.5   Auditory Training Methods

2.5.1   Auditory Training Theory

The auditory training is aimed to enlighten the children's auditory system. The auditory enlightenment method was performed following the normal children's hearing and language development regulation and the characteristics of children's development. And sounds should be given according to the development characteristics of the child. If the sound is given quickly, it will stop before the child is alert. Especially for children with profound hearing loss, it is difficult to recognize relatively short sounds, performance of recognizing continuous short-term sounds with short stimulation intervals is not good. So, when giving sounds, adjust gradually from slow to fast, long to short, to make children have a process of perceiving and adapting to sounds, become sensitive to the sound, and spontaneously search for the sound to complete tests accurately.

2.5.2 Strategies of Auditory Enlightenment

Initially understand the children's clinical hearing assessments and general conditions before and after birth, and observe the current physical growth and neuropsychological development of infants and young children. With the simultaneous use of hearing, sight, touch, and somatosensory stimulate the development of auditory cortex induction and movement and train children's pre-linguistic skills such as voice response, discrimination, and concept building, the detailed procedures are as follows:

- Keep the air in the training room fresh, with a temperature of 20–22 °C and humidity of 55–60% and ventilation every day. Understand children's physical growth, neuropsychological development and nurturing environment systematically, establish friendly feelings with children, and make them feel safe, take care of children before training, and keep them sleeping enough.
- Take the method of simultaneous multisensory stimulation and train the subjects' cerebral cortex induction and motor development systematically, build their skills such as sound perception, discrimination, and language development. In the beginning, take the form of one-to-one or two-to-one, 5 times a week, and 0.5–1 hour each time in the beginning, then 2 hours each time after the child is emotionally stable. The training mainly takes nurses as the principal part, and cultivates the detection and perception ability of infants and young children during play. Firstly, guide the children to take a look, touch, knock, and pinch, so that the children will be happy and gradually adapt to the environment; with the combination of audio–visual→visual–audio→audio–visual–audio, naked ears first and then wear a hearing aid and observe whether the child responds to the sound. After giving the sound, there must be sufficient time to wait for the response. The interval between the two sounds should be long, music should be tapped, the voice input time should be long enough, so that the child has a sufficient response process, adjust the distance of voice at any time, and conduct regular assessments and evaluations.
- Music→tone→speech and other sounds are given alternately and intermittently to help children perceive the existence of sound one by one.
- *Training mode*: Simultaneous participation of multiple senses such as vision, hearing, and touch. Visual stimulation uses picture observation response training to cultivate attention. The size of figure is 15 cm with different colors, there are 10 pictures each time and three times in total. Choose the figure according to age characteristics and choose test time according to the children's hobby. Auditory stimulation is carried out by listening to the sound first then fetching the toys. When giving sound, firstly there is no visual participation, and observe child's

reaction. If there is no response, use a combination of visual and auditory stimuli, and the loudness and distance of sound depend on the condition of child. Pay attention to the change of time when giving sound to avoid forming regularity. After giving sound, wait patiently for the child's response, observe the true situation of the child's perception of voice and identify whether the child cannot cooperate, or the sound is not heard. Give sounds to babies 5–12 months after birth and guide them to find the sound source, such as watching a light box or sounding objects to help form a second conditional emission. Tactile stimulation uses sound vibration to stimulate the limbs of children, and they can perceive the presence of sound through touch.

- *Exercise-assisted training*: Infants without enlarged vestibular aqueduct crawl and roll twice a day to promote the motor development of children with motor development retardation. Functional training is carried out in accordance with the law of motor development of children.
- Auditory training cases results.

Table 2.2 lists the hearing improvement with behavior observation audiometry of 7 children in our center after hearing training. It showed that some children have no response to sound with naked ears at first, and gradually complete the pediatric

Table 2.2 Behavior observation audiometry before and after training

Case	Training time	Age (m)	Side	250 Hz	500 Hz	1000 Hz	2000 Hz	4000 Hz
1	Pre.	22	L	/	/	/	/	/
	7 m po.			/	/	115	/	/
	9 m po.			110	115	105	115	/
2	Pre.	18	R	/	/	/	/	/
	4 m po.			/	/	/	/	/
	7 m po.			/	110	110	/	/
3	Pre.	18	L	/	/	/	/	/
	4 m po.			/	/	/	/	/
	7 m po.			110	115	115	115	/
4	Pre.	7	R	/	/	/	/	/
	4 m po.			110	110	115	115	115
	6 m po.			80	80	50	95	95
5	Pre.	6	L	/	/	/	/	/
	2 m po.			/	75	70	60	65
	4 m po.			90	80	65	60	70
6	Pre.	8	R	/	/	/	/	/
	3 m po.			100	105	105	/	/
7	Pre.	10	R	/	/	/	/	/
	3 m po.			/	/	/	/	/
	7 m po.			/	115	/	/	/
	10 m po.			/	95	110	/	/
	15 m po.			/	90	90	115	/
	21 m po.			/	95	95	/	/

m = month, pre. =pre-training; po. =post-training

behavior observation audiometry after training and the response time range from 2 to 7 months. The hearing curve gradually appears, it manifests as a reaction at a different frequency, or an increase at the original frequency. The results confirmed that with early hearing input, no matter how poor the residual hearing of children, they may benefit from auditory stimulation.

2.6 Conclusion

Before CI surgery, objective and subjective hearing test methods should be performed to determine the patients' residual hearing. The CCD patients' preoperative residual hearings are often poor, and when the objective and subjective hearing tests cannot be elicited, the auditory training before CI surgery is a good method to determine whether the patient's auditory pathway is integrity. The main purpose of auditory training is to awaken children's auditory perception ability, which includes the ability to detect changes in frequency, intensity, and duration. If after training the patients can observe hearing performance, it can give us the confidence of CI surgery.

References

Mason SM, O'Donoghue GM, et al. Perioperative electrical auditory brain stem response in candidates for pediatric cochlear implantation. Otol Neurotol. 1997;18:466–471.

Nikolopoulos TP, Mason SM, et al. The prognostic value of promontory electric auditory brain stem response in pediatric cochlear implantation. Ear Hear. 2000;21(3):236–41.

Shi Y, Chen B, et al. Transmastoidslotted labyrinthotomy approach cochlear implantation with customized electrode for patients with common cavity deformity. Zhonghua Er Bi Yan Hou Tou Jing Wai Ke Za Zhi. 2019 Jul 7;54(7):489–94.

Wei X, Li Y, et al. Slotted labyrinthotomy approach with customized electrode for patients with common cavity deformity. Laryngoscope. 2018;128(2):468–472.

Xia J, Wang W, et al. Cochlear implantation in 21 patients with common cavity malformation. Acta Otolaryngol. 2015;135(5):459–65.

Radiological Aspect of Common Cavity Deformity

3

Anandhan Dhanasingh, Xingmei Wei, Huaiyu Zhang,
Junfang Xian, Lifang Zhang, and Biao Chen

3.1 Introduction

Radiological imaging and the accurate identification of the anatomical structures from the affected inner ear plays an integral role in the clinical evaluation of sensorineural hearing loss (Aschendorff et al. 2011). A profound understanding of the inner ear anatomy is essential in the identification of the malformation types, in the selection of cochlear implant electrode array and in the surgical planning of placing the electrode array inside the cochlea. Knowing what to visualize from the clinical images in different viewing planes is essential in the identification of inner ear malformation types. It could be mentally challenging in compiling the series of CT image slices to bring a threedimensional (3D) representation of the anatomical structure (Dhanasingh et al. 2019). The ultimate aim of the imaging evaluation is to make a clinical decision whether to place the CI electrode into the inner ear or not.

The original version of this chapter was revised. The correction to this chapter can be found at https://doi.org/10.1007/978-981-16-8217-9_11

A. Dhanasingh (✉)
MED-EL Medical Electronics GmbH, Innsbruck, Austria
e-mail: Anandhan.Dhanasingh@medel.com

X. Wei · L. Zhang · B. Chen
Department of Otorhinolaryngology Head and Neck Surgery, Beijing Tongren Hospital, Capital Medical University, Beijing, China

Key Laboratory of Otolaryngology Head and Neck Surgery (Capital Medical University), Ministry of Education, Beijing, China

H. Zhang · J. Xian
Department of Radiology, Beijing Tongren Hospital, Capital Medical University, Beijing, China

© The Author(s), under exclusive license to Springer Nature Singapore Pte Ltd. 2022, corrected publication 2022
Y. Li (ed.), *Cochlear Implantation for Common Cavity Deformity*,
https://doi.org/10.1007/978-981-16-8217-9_3

This chapter will walk you through how common cavity (CC) is visualized in the preoperative clinical imaging in different planes and the importance of intra- and postoperative imaging in quality control of the CI electrode placement. Also, a method of visualizing the CC in 3D is discussed.

3.2   The Role of Imaging in Common Cavity Deformity

Computed Tomography (CT) and Magnetic Resonance Imaging (MRI) are complementary in the preoperative analysis of the inner ear malformation. High-resolution CT in particular enables visualizing the bony structures, osseous details as well as variant anatomy of the inner ear, whereas the MRI is essential in the assessment of the auditory nerve (Bhagat et al. 2020). CT comes up with the concern of radiation dose, especially in the pediatrics, but the newer cone-beam techniques offer enhanced imaging resolution at relatively lower radiation doses compared to traditional multi-detector CT. High-resolution, 3D T_2W (T_2 weighted) images on MRI with a special resolution of 0.4 mm enable visualizing neural structures (Quirk et al. 2019).

3.2.1   Common Cavity in CT

Knowing how a normal anatomy inner ear would look like in clinical imaging in different planes, would certainly help to identify the inner ear malformation types. In the axial view of the normal anatomy inner ear, the line drawn parallel to the internal auditory canal (IAC) separates the cochlear and the vestibular portion (Weiss et al. 2021). The basal, middle, and apical turn of the cochlea is well distinguishable, and the lateral semicircular canal of the vestibular part is also seen. The classic common cavity, as per the definition, is a single cavity that represents both the cochlear and the vestibular portions with no inter-scala septum separating the turns of the cochlea. The vestibular portion may or may not have semicircular canals. The white line drawn parallel to the IAC still distinguishes the cochlear and the vestibular portion. The cochlear aplasia with the presence of a vestibular cavity is well distinguishable from the classic common cavity (Weiss et al. 2021). The white line drawn parallel to the IAC shows only the vestibular cavity under the line with no cochlear portion seen above the line. In the oblique coronal plane, the normal anatomy inner ear shows the basal turn of the cochlea along with the three semicircular canals. However, the classic common cavity and the cochlear aplasia with the vestibular cavity, are seen as a single cavity as shown in Fig. 3.1 lower panel.

The two-dimensional (2D) images do show the anatomical structures provided if the image readers are experienced enough to understand the anatomy. Visualizing the inner ear in 3D adds additional perspective and could make the understanding of the anatomy lot easier. 3D segmentation of the inner ear from the preoperative DICOM images is described elsewhere by Dhanasingh et al. (2019). Briefly, the image data sets were loaded into 3D slicer freeware (3D Slicer, https://www.slicer.org/; version 4.8.0) followed by segmentation of the complete inner ear structures including the IAC. Axial plane is better suitable for the segmentation of these

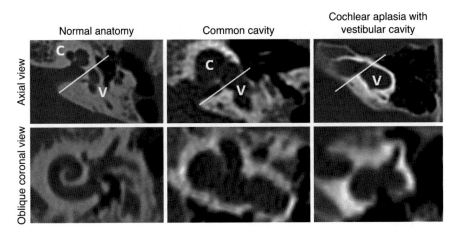

Fig. 3.1 Comparison of normal anatomy inner ear with classic common cavity and cochlear aplasia with a vestibular cavity

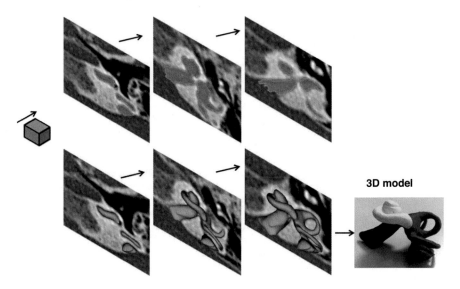

Fig. 3.2 Segmentation of the inner ear from every image slice available in the image dataset. Summing up all the segmented images transforms into a 3D model (reproduced from Dhanasingh A. Variations in the Size and Shape of Human Cochlear Malformation Types. Anat Rec (Hoboken) 2019, 302(10):1792–1799)

structures by setting a tight grayscale threshold to avoid capturing undesired structures (refer Fig. 3.2). Figure 3.2 elaborates the segmentation process. Approximately 10 minutes is needed to segment the complete inner ear including the IAC from clinical imaging dataset.

It is important to visualize the anatomical structures of interest from all possible views because some structures are only visible in one particular plane and not visible in the other planes. Figure 3.3 shows some of the vestibular cavity cases received

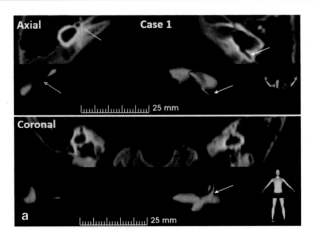

Fig. 3.3 Cases of vestibular cavity showing the presence and absence of SCC and the connection between the IAC and the cavity. The size of the cavity itself is seen varying in size and shape. (**a**) The axial view shows lateral SCC (white arrow). Right side shows a disconnection between the IAC and the cavity (yellow arrow). The coronal view shows the anterior SCC (white). Red arrow points to the very small cochlear portion/ anteroinferior portion of the cavity. The size of the cavity is seen as smaller on the right side compared to the left side. (**b**) The axial view shows no presence of semicircular canals. The yellow arrow points to very narrow connection between the IAC and the cavity. The white arrow in the coronal view shows the presence of anterior SCC on both sides and the red arrow points to the anteroinferior position of the cavity. The left side cavity is seen smaller compared to the right side. (**c**) The axial view shows a narrow connection between IAC and the cavity on both sides (*yellow arrow*). In the 2D image, there is no visibility of the lateral SCC whereas the 3D images clearly show its presence (*white arrow*). The coronal view shows the presence of anterior SCC (*white arrow*) and the red arrow points to the anteroinferior position of the cavity. (**d**) The axial view shows a narrow connection between the IAC and the cavity on the left side. The white arrow points to the lateral SCC. In the coronal plane, anterior SCC is visible on both sides as pointed by the white arrow. The red arrow points to the anteroinferior portion of the cavity and the right side shows a better developed cochlear portion. (**e**) The axial view shows a clear presence of lateral SCC (*white arrow*) and the yellow arrow points to the missing connection between the IAC and the cavity. In the coronal plane, anterior SCC is visible as pointed by the white arrow and the red arrow points to the doubtful anteroinferior portion of the cavity that represents the auditory function. (**f**) The axial view shows a very doubtful connection between IAC and the cavity. The coronal view shows the presence of anterior SCC as pointed by the white arrow and the anteroinferior portion on both sides by the red arrow. The left side cavity is seen smaller in size compared to the right side. (**g**) The axial view shows a doubtful connection between the IAC and the cavity on both sides are pointed by the yellow arrow. The white arrow points to the lateral SCC. In the coronal view, the white arrow points to the anterior SCC and the red arrow points to the anteroinferior portion of the cavity

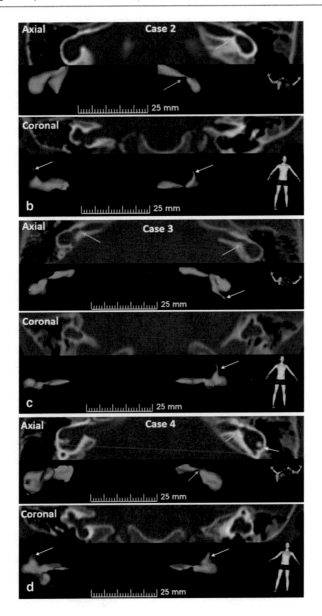

Fig. 3.3 (continued)

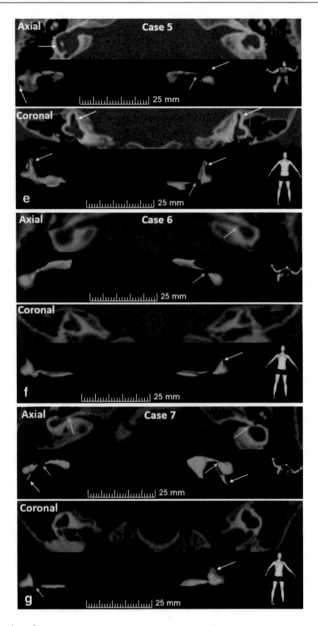

Fig. 3.3 (continued)

from across the world in both axial and coronal views. It catches most of the variation in its size, shape, and the presence of anatomical structures. The white arrow points to the semicircular canals (SCC), the yellow arrow points to the connection between IAC and the cavity and the red arrow points to the anteroinferior portion of the cavity that is believed to carry the auditory neural elements (Yamazaki et al. 2014).

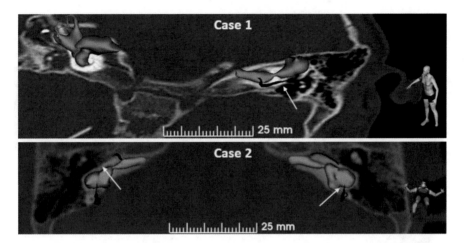

Fig. 3.4 3D segmentation of the inner ear showing the cavity and the course of the facial nerve. Case 1 is in oblique plane and case 2 is in axial plane. The white arrow points to the facial nerve

Figure 3.3 is an example that shows the size, shape, and anatomical structures are highly variable within this malformation type and every case has to be analyzed individually to understand the anatomy before the CI surgery. Absence of a prominent connection between the IAC and the cavity should be dealt carefully. Assessment tool like promontory electric stimulation followed by a recording of eABR responses is one way of assessing the potency of the nerve in carrying electric stimulation from the cavity to the auditory cortex (Polterauer et al. 2018). Auditory brainstem implant (ABI) is another option, in case of the assessment tool fails to find any useful eABR or even CI fails to produce meaningful hearing outcomes.

Finding the course of facial nerve starting from the IAC till it crosses the cavity is important as this will help in the surgical planning of placing the electrode without harming the facial nerve. Literature has reported on the aberrant course of facial nerve crossing the path of electrode insertion (Song et al. 2012). Figure 3.4 shows two cases with cavity representing the vestibular portion of the inner ear and the course of the facial nerve. It might be highly difficult to mentally bring in the picture of facial nerve just by looking at the 2D images. The 3D segmentation makes it easy to visualize the complete course of facial nerve from the IAC till it crosses the cavity.

3.2.2 MRI in Visualizing the Nerve Structure in the IAC

Within the CI application, magnetic resonance imaging (MRI), especially heavily T2-weighted sequences are clinically used in analyzing the presence of nerves that run through the IAC (Young et al. 2012). In a normal anatomy inner ear, a cross section through the IAC in the sagittal oblique plane as shown in Fig. 3.5a, yellow dotted line, would show two prominent dots representing facial (VII) on the left and cochlear-vestibular nerve (CVN) on the right. A cross-section bit closer to the cochlea as shown by the red dotted line in Fig. 3.5a, would show four prominent

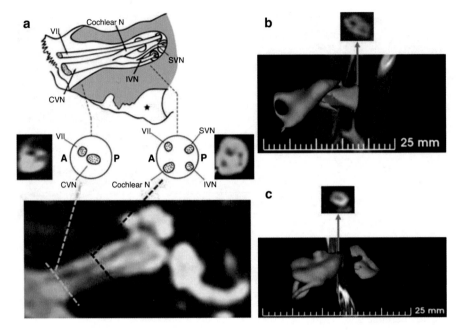

Fig. 3.5 Cross-sectional (c/s) view of the IAC showing the nerve bundles. Normal anatomy cochlea shows four prominent dots in the c/s of IAC close to the cochlea representing facial nerve (VII), cochlear nerve, superior (SVN) and inferior vestibular nerve (IVN) (**a**) Sample 1 of CC shows two prominent dots in the c/s of IAC (reproduced with permission from Young et al. 2012) (**b**) Sample 2 of CC showing one elliptical dot in the c/s of IAC (**c**)

dots. The dot at the top left corner is the facial nerve, bottom left corner has the cochlear nerve and the top and bottom corners at the right side represent the nerves connecting the superior and the inferior portion of the vestibular organ, respectively.

Two samples of CC in our collection had MRI and the cross section through the IAC showed two prominent dots in one sample (Fig. 3.5b) and one elongated elliptical dot in the other sample (Fig. 3.5c). The question of whether the nerve fibers corresponding to the cochlear portion is present or not in the nerve bundle, is open and is discussed in detail under the chapter "Electrode design and optimal placement section."

3.3 Importance of Intra- and/or Postoperative Imaging in CC

One of the well-documented complications with electrode insertion in CC malformation type is the electrode entering the IAC (Aschendorff 2011). The electrode design along with the surgical technique plays a major role in this complication.

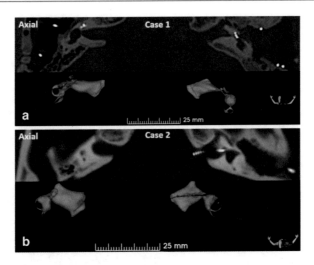

Fig. 3.6 Post-operative image of two cases showing the presence of straight electrode in the IAC. (**a**) Left side shows a vestibular cavity with a straight electrode implanted but wrongly placed almost into the IAC. The stimulating channels are nowhere closer to the periphery of the cavity. (**b**) Left side shows a clear absence of the cochlear portion with the cavity representing the vestibular portion. The straight electrode is wrongly placed completely inside the IAC

Figure 3.6 showcases two cases of cavity representing the vestibular portion with the electrode placed inside the IAC, which needed revision surgery later in correcting it. The surgical approach of electrode insertion in these two cases is through the traditional facial recess approach (TFRA) that offered no chance for the electrode to make a nice loop inside the cavity. This situation could have been avoided if the intraoperative imaging would have done. Intraoperative imaging is highly recommended in difficult cases to quality check the proper placement of the electrode inside the cavity. If found electrode in the IAC, it can be corrected in the same surgery without placing the patient at risk of inviting them for a revision surgery later.

Figure 3.7 showcases three cases from China one case from Italy that were implanted with customized electrode design (red structure) from MED-EL that shows some portion of the electrode contacts placed closer proximity to the antero-inferior (AI) location. The flexible nature of the electrode array along with the Transmastoid Slotted Labyrinthotomy Approach (TSLA) as proposed by Beltrame et al. (2000) and Wei et al. in 2018 is essential in the optimal placement of the electrode in the AI location. The postoperative imaging is highly useful in finding the electrode contacts that are closer to the anteroinferior location of the cavity where it is believed to have the auditory nerve fibers as pointed by white arrows in Fig. 3.7. Also, the postoperative imaging is useful in identifying the electrode channels that are placed outside the cavity and deactivating them thereby eliminating nonauditory sensation.

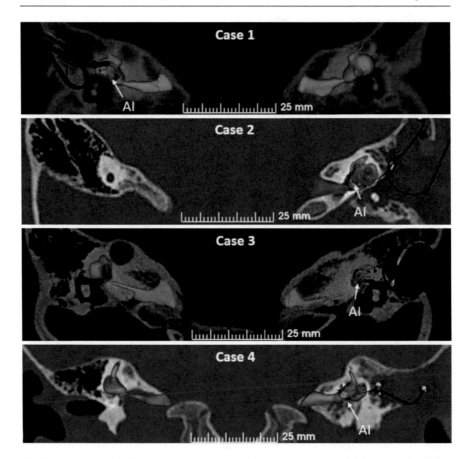

Fig. 3.7 Postoperative 3D segmented inner ear of four cases implanted with the customized electrode design from MED-EL showing the electrodes in the anteroinferior (AI) location

3.4   Correlation between Radiological Findings and CI Outcomes

Prof. Yongxin Li's team from the Beijing Tongren hospital, in China, evaluated the relationship between radiological findings and CI outcomes from twenty CCD patients. This section reports the correlation between the CI outcomes as evaluated by Categories of Auditory Performance (CAP) and the volume of the cavity as calculated by the advanced DICOM viewer.

The volume of the 3D segmented cavity was measured by the 3D slicer (advanced DICOM viewer) software as shown in Fig. 3.8. The volume of the cavity from 20 patients is given in Table within Fig. 3.8 and it ranges from 12.21 mm³ to 292.96 mm³.

A CAP score of 4 points is a critical value that usually corresponds to the ability of patients to discriminate sound without lip reading. It takes a certain time for the patient to reach the CAP score of 4 points and in this study, the cavity volume was

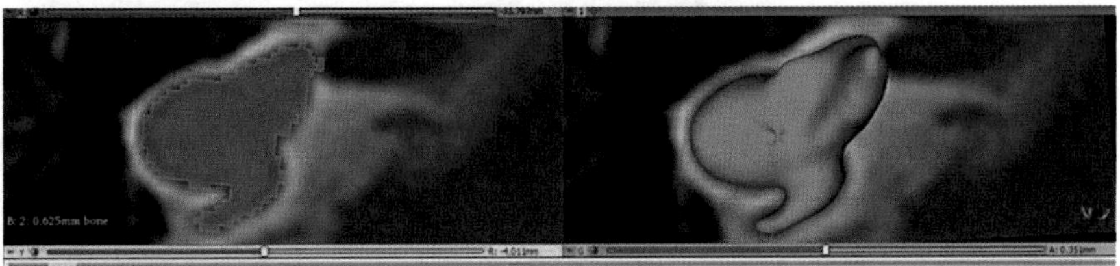

A	B	C	D
1 Segment	Number of voxels [voxels] (1)	Volume [mm3] (1)	Volume [cm3] (1)
2 Segment_1 4664		179.856	0.179856

Fig. 3.8 Measurement of the cavity volume in 3D slicer (advanced DICOM viewer)

correlated to the time at which the patients reached the CAP score of 4 points. Patients with cavity volume > 141.78 mm^3 took between 18.11 and 23.03 months with an average time of 20.57 months to reach the critical CAP score. Whereas the patients with cavity volume < 141.78 mm^3 took only 8.39–14.86 months with an average time of 11.63 months to reach the critical CAP score. The difference between the two groups was statistically significant ($p = 0.02$). The trend was toward patients with smaller cavity volumes reaching the critical CAP score faster than the patients with bigger cavity volume. The only explanation that can be given here is the smaller cavity will have more surface area to be covered with the electrode contacts enabling effective stimulation of the neuronal elements, compared to the bigger cavity.

3.5 Multiplanar Volume Rendering (MPVR) Technique in the Assessment of Electrode Location and CI Outcomes

Prof. Yongxin Li's research team and radiology department from the Beijing Tongren hospital, in China, are currently evaluating the relationship between the distance from each electrode to the cavity wall and the hearing outcomes. 3D segmentation of the cavity and the electrodes were performed using the multiplanar volume rendered (MPVR) (Fig. 3.9). From the 3D model, the individual electrode channels were identified, and the corresponding image slices were used in measuring the distance between the center of the electrode contact to the wall cavity (Fig. 3.10). The preliminary results evaluated from 25 patients with CC deformity implanted with CI revealed that maximum comfort level (MCL) in the audio processor fitting was lower and better audiological outcomes were associated in cases with shorter distances between the electrode and the cavity wall. This conveys the message that the optimal location for the electrode inside the cavity is close to the cavity wall where the neuronal elements are believed to be present.

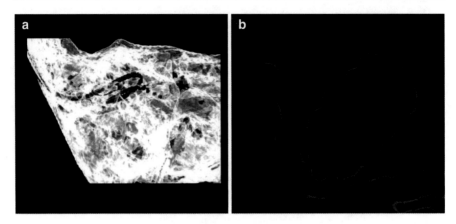

Fig. 3.9 The procedure of multiplanar volume reconstruction (MPVR) technique for CCD after CI. (**a**) The VR image of electrode and temporal bone and (**b**) MPVR images were reconstructed and the layer of electrode's middle level was selected to measure the distance (reproduced with permission from Wei et al. 2022, Front. Neurol. 12:783225)

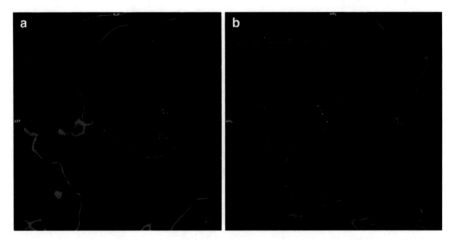

Fig. 3.10 Measurement of distance between electrode and cavity wall. (**a**) The method of evaluation of the distance between the electrode and cavity wall in situations involving the fusion of the silica gel sleeve outside the electrode and wall of the common cavity and (**b**) The method of evaluation of the distance between the electrode and cavity wall in scenarios that do not involve fusion of the silica gel sleeve and cavity wall (reproduced with permission from Wei et al. 2022, Front. Neurol. 12:783225)

3.6   Conclusion

Imaging, in general, is an invaluable tool in the identification of anatomical structures of interest before, during, or after the surgery. While 2D image slicers are good enough to understand the anatomical structures and this comes with a learning curve, visualizing in 3D is much easier in understanding the anatomical structures in a quick time. Spending additional ten minutes in 3D segmenting the complete inner ear would prove worth avoiding several complications. Intraoperative/postoperative imaging is very useful in quality checking the proper placement of the electrode inside the cavity as well as in identifying the electrode contacts that are closer to the anteroinferior location of the cavity. Measuring the cavity volume would give an approximate time at which the patient might reach the critical CAP score. Overall, a good preoperative analysis of the imaging could avoid several complications later on and could predict the audiological outcomes.

References

Aschendorff A. Imaging in cochlear implant patients. GMS curr top Otorhinolaryngol. Head Neck Surg. 2011;10:Doc07.

Beltrame MA, Bonfioli F, Frau GN. Cochlear implant in inner ear malformation: double posterior labyrinthotomy approach to common cavity. Adv Otorhinolaryngol. 2000;57:113–9.

Bhagat AC, Kumar J, Garg A, Prakash A, Meher R, Arya S. Imaging in congenital inner ear malformations-an algorithmic approach. Indian J Radiol. Imaging. 2020 Apr–Jun;30(2):139–48.

Dhanasingh A. Variations in the size and shape of human Cochlear malformation types. Anat Rec (Hoboken). 2019 Oct;302(10):1792–9.

Dhanasingh A, Dietz A, Jolly C, Roland P. Human inner-ear malformation types captured in 3D. J Int Adv Otol. 2019 Apr;15(1):77–82.

Polterauer D, Mandruzatto G, Neuling M, Polak M, Müller J, John-Martin H. PromBERA: a preoperative eABR: an update. Curr Dir Biomed Eng. 2018;4:563–5.

Quirk B, Youssef A, Ganau M, D'Arco F. Radiological diagnosis of the inner ear malformations in children with sensorineural hearing loss. BJR Open. 2019 Jun 14;1(1):20180050.

Song JJ, Park JH, Jang JH, Lee JH, Oh SH, Chang SO, Kim CS. Facial nerve aberrations encountered during cochlear implantation. Acta Otolaryngol. 2012 Jul;132(7):788–94.

Wei X, Li Y, Fu QJ, Gong Y, Chen B, Chen J, Shi Y, Su Q, Cui D, Liu T. Slotted labyrinthotomy approach with customized electrode for patients with common cavity deformity. Laryngoscope. 2018 Feb;128(2):468–72.

Weiss NM, Langner S, Mlynski R, Roland P, Dhanasingh A. Evaluating Common Cavity Cochlear Deformities Using CT Images and 3D Reconstruction. Laryngoscope. 2021 Feb;131(2):386–391.

Yamazaki H, Naito Y, Fujiwara K, Moroto S, Yamamoto R, Yamazaki T, Sasaki I. Electrically evoked auditory brainstem response-based evaluation of the spatial distribution of auditory neuronal tissue in common cavity deformities. Otol Neurotol. 2014 Sep;35(8):1394–402.

Young NM, Kim FM, Ryan ME, Tournis E, Yaras S. Pediatric cochlear implantation of children with eighth nerve deficiency. Int J Pediatr Otorhinolaryngol. 2012 Oct;76(10):1442–8.

Electrode Array Design and Surgical Technique in Common Cavity Deformity

4

Anandhan Dhanasingh

4.1   Introduction

One of the key determinants of cochlear implantation (CI) success lies in the effective placement of the electrode array inside the cochlea in closer proximity to the neural elements (Dhanasingh and Jolly 2017). This becomes even more important when comes to the inner ear with abnormal anatomy like common cavity (CC) (Wei et al. 2018; Yamazaki et al. 2014). A good understanding of the CC anatomy is important in bringing the stimulating electrode contacts close to the neural elements. The electrodes that are in current clinical application varies a lot in its size, shape, and contact orientation, and a good understanding of the electrode design would help the clinicians in choosing the best suitable electrode matching the CC size, shape, and anatomy (Dhanasingh and Jolly 2017; Beltrame et al. 2013). The surgical placement of the electrode inside the CC depends on the CC anatomy and the electrode design chosen. Literature has evidenced several cases of CC in which electrodes have been misplaced and revision surgery was performed to correct it (Bloom et al. 2009). This chapter will describe the advantages and disadvantages of the current clinical use electrode designs in CC. This section will also showcase customized electrode designs for CC of different sizes. Surgical placement of every electrode designs that are in clinical use will also be covered in detail.

The original version of this chapter was revised. The correction to this chapter can be found at
https://doi.org/10.1007/978-981-16-8217-9_11

A. Dhanasingh (✉)
MED-EL Medical Electronics GmbH, Innsbruck, Austria
e-mail: Anandhan.Dhanasingh@medel.com

© The Author(s), under exclusive license to Springer Nature
Singapore Pte Ltd. 2022, corrected publication 2022
Y. Li (ed.), *Cochlear Implantation for Common Cavity Deformity*,
https://doi.org/10.1007/978-981-16-8217-9_4

4.2   Anatomy of Common Cavity

From the embryological explanation, the CC is the result of disruption in the dif-ferentiation of inner ear structures during the 4th and 5th week of gestation (Cock 1838; Yiin et al. 2011). At this time of gestation, the entire inner ear appears in the form of a single cavity representing both the cochlear and the vestibular portion. This single cavity is called a classic CC as shown in Fig. 4.1(b). In a normal

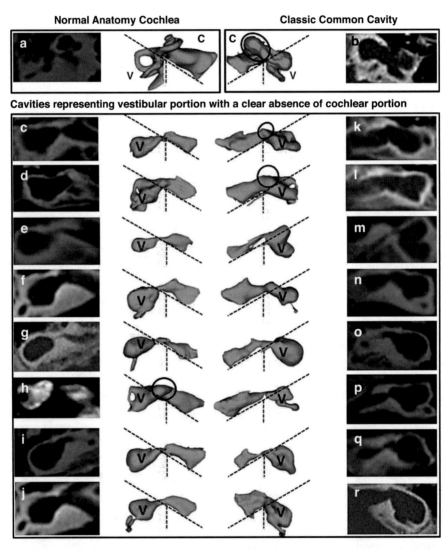

Fig. 4.1 Samples of cochlea seen in its axial view both in two- and in three-dimensional. Normal anatomy cochlea with the black dotted line parallel to the internal auditory canal separating the cochlear (C) and the vestibular (V) portion (**a**). The classic common cavity shows the cochlear and the vestibular portions separated by the black dotted line drawn parallel to the internal auditory canal (IAC) (**b**). Samples C-R are from patients across the world that show the cavity that repre-sents the vestibular portion with a clear absence of the cochlear portion

anatomy cochlea seen its axial view, a straight line is drawn parallel to the internal auditory canal (IAC) as shown in Fig. 4.1(a) would separate the cochlear and the vestibular portion (Weiss et al. 2021). The same thing holds true in the classic CC as well as shown in Fig. 4.1(b). However, several cases (Fig. 4.1 C-R), which are mistakenly called as classic CC by clinicians across the world, are actually not classic CC but the cavity representing the vestibular portion with a clear absence of the cochlear portion (Beltrame et al. 2005; Mylanus et al. 2004; Manolidis et al. 2006; Kimura et al. 2017; Sennaroglu et al. 2006). Still, these cases are implanted with CI and have been reported with varying degrees of hearing performance. The anatomy of the cavities (C-R) shows a huge variation overall in the structures present, size, and the shape of the cavity, with some samples shown in Fig. 4.1 (C, E, I, and O) showing a clear absence of the semicircular canals (SCC) whereas samples in Fig. 4.1 (D, F, G, H, J, K, L, M, N, P, Q, and R) show some form of SCC development.

4.3   Geometry of CC

Qualitatively looking at Fig. 4.1, the size of the CC is seen as highly variable and the CC in most of the cases assumes an elliptical shape. The length of the long and short axes of the elliptical cavity is measured in the axial view as shown in Fig. 4.2.

Calculating the circumference of the ellipse is one way of measuring the CC size and it is helpful in the selection of the electrode array length. The circumference of the ellipse can be calculated using Raman's equation ($2\pi \sqrt{((a^2 + b^2)/2)}$), where a and b are half the length of long axis and short axis, respectively. Figure 4.3(a and b) shows a plot between the long axis and short axis length versus the calculated circumference of the cavity of sixteen samples shown in Fig. 4.1. From these samples, we found that the long axis length varies from a minimum of 5 mm to a maximum of 13.5 mm and the short axis length varies from a minimum of 3 mm to a maximum of 8 mm. Accordingly, the circumference of the cavity varied from a minimum of 15 mm to a maximum of 30 mm requiring electrode array lengths between 15 and 30 mm.

Fig. 4.2 CC visualized in the axial plane with the measurement of long axis and short axis length

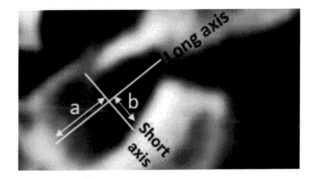

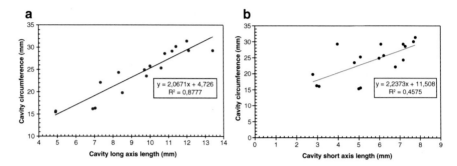

Fig. 4.3 Plot between long-axis length (**a**) and short-axis length (**b**) versus the calculated circumference of the cavity

Fig. 4.4 Axial view of a vestibular cavity with the depiction of neural elements extending from the IAC along the periphery of the cavity

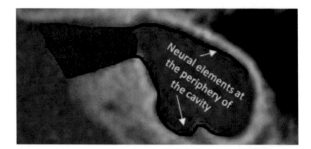

4.4 Neuroanatomy of CC

The cavity is normally filled with cochlear fluid with no visible structures inside. The cochlear–vestibular neuroepithelium is present at the periphery of the cavity which are the extensions from the IAC as shown in Fig. 4.4 by the red-colored illustration. The neural fibers from the IAC are believed to sprout out along the periphery of the cavity. In order to stimulate these neural elements effectively, the electrode should be implanted with the contact pads facing toward the neural elements (Graham et al. 2000; McElveen et al. 1997).

4.5 Electrode Insertion Complications with CC

The CC malformation type lacks the cochlear lumen as seen in normal anatomy cochlea in which placing a regular CI electrode array is straightforward. The CC as seen surgically after opening the mastoid is the lateral end of the cavity and the IAC is somewhat in-line with the surgical view as shown in Fig. 4.5. This increases the chances of any electrode type entering the IAC, when it is intended to be placed inside the cavity with the insertion angle in-line with the IAC.

Literature has evidenced incidences of electrode entering the IAC which has been identified by either intraoperative or postoperative images and needed revision

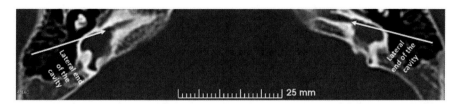

Fig. 4.5 CC seen in the axial view with the white arrow marks pointing to the IAC which is in-line with the surgical view from the mastoid surface

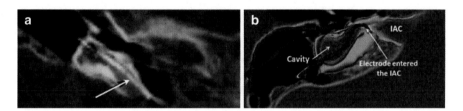

Fig. 4.6 Intraoperative image showing the presence of electrode array inside the IAC in a case of CC (**a**) (Bloom et al. 2009). 3D segmented from the postoperative image showing the electrode entered the IAC in a case of CC (**b**)

surgery to correct it (Bloom et al. 2009). Not to forget that the IAC carries the nerve bundle and any disruption to those sensitive structures could disturb or prevent the electrical stimulation from the electrode to be carried to the auditory cortex. Figure 4.6 showcases two cases of such electrode entering the IAC that was identified from the intraoperative (Fig. 4.6a) and postoperative images (Fig. 4.6b).

A pre-curved modiolar hugging electrode may sound like a good choice in terms of easy implantation process. But the downside of this electrode type is that the stimulating contacts are facing the inner wall of the curvature whereas the CC lacks any central modiolus trunk and the neural elements are present at the periphery of the cavity wall. The other downside of this electrode type as a choice for CC is that the size and the shape of the pre-curved portion of this electrode are fixed at a diameter of approximately 5 mm as shown in Fig. 4.7a Whereas the size of the cavity is seen as highly variable as shown in Fig. 4.3. Figure 4.7b shows 3 different sizes of an ellipse and Fig. 4.7c shows the pre-curved electrode in those 3 different sized ellipses demonstrating different fitness between the elliptical size and the pre-curved electrode. The ellipse with the short axis length of 5 mm provides a good fit to pre-curved electrode (Fig. 4.7c middle) whereas for the ellipses with the short axis length of 8 and 3 mm provides a loose-fit if not, the cavity is too small to accommodate this electrode, respectively.

It is known from the literature that an electrode array that is floating away from the wall of the cavity would be expected to deliver low or fluctuating current levels, with less satisfactory implant performances. This fits the observation of Tucci et al. (1995) that in such cases the current levels produced by the implant may fluctuate. Intraoperative radiological imaging may be helpful in making sure that a straight

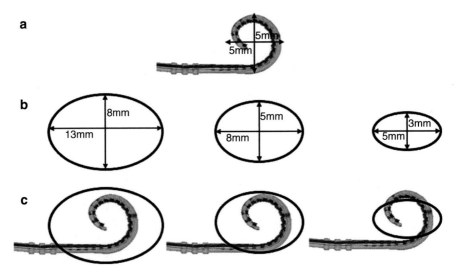

Fig. 4.7 Approximate diameter of the pre-curved portion of a commercially available modiolar hugging electrode (**a**). Three different sizes of an ellipse mimick the size variation of a CC (**b**). A single-sized modiolar hugging electrode in three different sized ellipses shows the mismatch between one-sized electrode and varying sized CC (**c**)

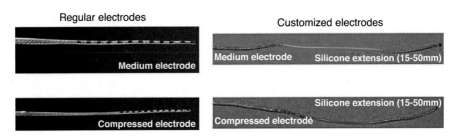

Fig. 4.8 MEDIUM and COMPRESSED electrode in the regular format and as well in the customized electrode format with the silicone extension

electrode array has adopted the curve of the cavity. A good understanding of the CC anatomy, how the IAC is positioned in relation to the cavity along with the intended angle of electrode insertion and on the electrode design itself, would avoid several complications post-surgery.

4.6 Customized Electrode Choice

The need for a customized electrode choice for the CC malformation type arises with the literature evidencing regular electrode entering the IAC as shown in Fig. 4.6. It was Prof. Beltrame from Italy in **1999** proposed a modified electrode array design that carries a silicone dummy extension at the tip of the active electrode array as shown in Fig. 4.8. It was through a scientific collaboration between Prof.

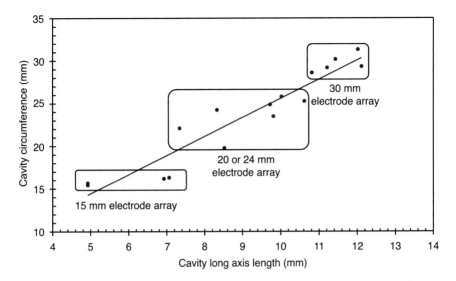

Fig. 4.9 A chart showing the electrode array length choice for the CC circumference. Below the chart given in the special electrode array design shows a silicone dummy extension connected to the tip of the electrode array

Beltrame and MED-EL, a CI manufacturer head-quartered in Austria designed and fabricated this customized electrode and is in clinical use since 1999.

With the size of the cavity seen highly varying, one length electrode array might not be a good strategy for CC. Figure 4.9 is a chart for the electrode array length selection matching the cavity circumference based on the cavity size measurement from the preoperative radiological image. A 15-mm long electrode array would be a good choice for the cavity circumference of around 15 mm to 20 mm. A 20- or 24-mm long electrode array can be safely chosen for the cavity circumference varying between 20 and 25 mm. A longer-length electrode array in the range of 30 mm would be a good choice for cavity circumference measuring anything above 27 mm. Upon a custom request from the operating surgeon, MED-EL, a CI manufacturer is able to custom fabricate the chosen electrode array length with the silicone extension attached to the electrode tip. By choosing the electrode array length matching the cavity size, the best electrode–cavity fit can be achieved.

4.7   Surgical Approach in Electrode Placement

Apart from the electrode design, the surgical approach plays a key role in the proper placement of the electrode array inside the cavity, avoiding all postsurgical complications.

Double posterior labyrinthotomy approach was proposed by Prof. Beltrame (Beltrame et al. 2000) as a new surgical approach for placing the customized electrode safely inside the cavity making sure the stimulating channels are placed close to the periphery of the cavity. His approach involves making two openings onto the lateral end of the cavity wall followed by inserting the tip of the electrode through one hole and pulling it out through the other hole as shown in Fig. 4.10. This will ensure the electrode array to form a nice loop inside the cavity with no chance of entering the IAC. Instead of two separate openings, it was also proposed to use a single slit labyrinthectomy, in the form of an elliptical opening, depending on the surgical ease.

The single slit labyrinthotomy for introducing the electrode inside the cavity was named as Transmastoid Slotted Labyrinthotomy Approach (TSLA) by Wei et al. in 2017. In parallel to this approach, Wei et al. also clinically applied the Traditional Facial Recess Approach (TFRA) for introducing the electrode into the cavity. They compared the two approaches of TSLA with the customized electrode design and TFRA with regular commercially available straight electrodes in six patients each for the surgical time and the hearing outcomes (Fig. 4.11). The results are given in Table 4.1.

The average surgical time for TFRA and TSLA approaches were 83.3 and 46.4 minutes, respectively. The recommended TSLA approach with the customized

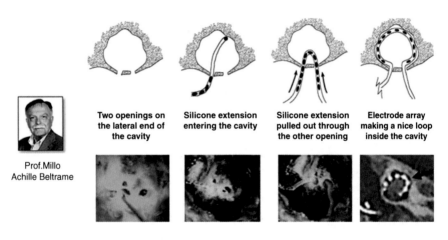

Prof. Millo
Achille Beltrame

| Two openings on the lateral end of the cavity | Silicone extension entering the cavity | Silicone extension pulled out through the other opening | Electrode array making a nice loop inside the cavity |

Fig. 4.10 Prof. Millo Achille Beltrame, an otorhinolaryngologist from Italy who proposed the customized electrode design and double posterior labyrinthotomy surgical approach for placing the electrode safely and effectively inside the cavity

Table 4.1 Surgical time and audiological outcomes between TFRA and TSLA approaches of electrode placement

Group	Surgical time (min)	CAP before/after CI	SIR before/after CI	MUSS	MAIS/ IT-MAIS
TFRA	83.3	0.5/2.4	0.8/1.8	4.6	5.2
TSLA	46.4	0.7/2.9	1.0/1.4	5.1	13.0

TFRA, Traditional Facial Recess Approach; TSLA, Transmastoid Slotted Labyrinthotomy Approach; CAP, Categories of Auditory Performance; SIR, Speech Intelligibility Rating; MUSS, Meaningful Use of Speech Scale; Combined score for the Meaningful Auditory Integration Scale/ Infant-Toddler and the Meaningful Auditory Integration Scale

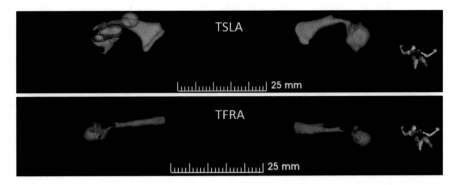

Fig. 4.11 Comparison between the TSLA and TFRA approach of electrode placement inside the cavity

electrode over the TFRA approach with a regular electrode, for that reason that TSLA offered a very stable electrode position within the cavity over a one-year follow-up time. The audiological outcomes were more favorable for the TSLA approach over TFRA approach and the supporting point for favoring the TSLA approach is the effective positioning of the electrode closer to the neuronal elements. The effective electrode position inside the cavity is detailed in the Sect. 4.8.

Electrode design, surgical procedure, and handling of the electrode play a key role in the optimal placement of the electrode inside the cavity.

4.8   Effective Location for Providing Electrical Stimulation Inside the Cavity

As seen in the normal anatomy inner ear in the axial view, the cochlear part is located anteriorly and slightly inferiorly as shown in Fig. 4.12, left side image. In a classic CC, the cochlear portion and the neural elements representing the auditory sensation are believed to be present in the anteroinferior portion of the cavity as shown in Fig. 4.12, middle image. The cavity that represents the vestibular portion only as shown in Fig. 4.12, right side image, the portion that is marked by the red circle, which is in the anterior portion, is where the neural elements representing auditory sensation are believed to be present (Yamazaki et al. 2014).

In 2014, Dr. Yamazaki and colleagues from Kobe city medical center general hospital in Japan investigated the spatial distribution of auditory neuronal tissue in CC deformity using electrically evoked brainstem response (eABR) during cochlear implantation (Yamazaki et al. 2014). Figure 4.13 is a recreation from their work that shows a case of CC in the coronal plane with the anteroinferior (AI) location marked by the red circle. This is the location where the neural fibers representing auditory sensation are believed to be present. In the first implantation (before re-implantation), the electrode array, in particular, Channel 19 and Channel 17 that are proximate to the anteroinferior location are a bit away from the periphery of the cavity. A weak

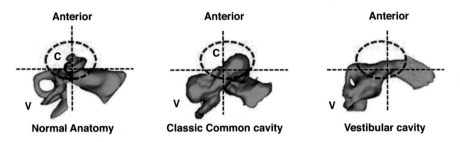

Fig. 4.12 Axial view of normal anatomy inner ear, classic common cavity, and cavity representing vestibular portion. Normal anatomy inner ear with the cochlear portion in the anterior location inside the red dotted circle (*left side image*). Classic common cavity with the cochlear portion of the cavity in the anterior location inside the red dotted circle (*central image*). Cavity represents vestibular portion with a tiny bud-like cochlear portion along the anterior location inside the red dotted circle (*right side image*)

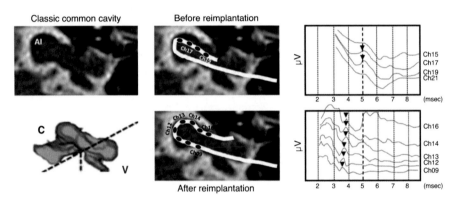

Fig. 4.13 A case of classic CC seen in the axial view with the anteroinferior (AI) location marked by the red circle. Post-op image of the first-time implantation showing the electrode (Channels 17 and 19) bit away from the AI location and its corresponding wave V of eABR at a latency of 5 ms. After reimplantation in re-positioning the electrode much closer to the AI location, the wave V of eABR were seen much prominently and at a shorter latency of 3.8 ms

wave V of the eABR was seen at a latency of 5 ms which is slightly longer in comparison to the cochlea without any inner-ear malformation. This case underwent re-implantation with a wide opening (3 mm diameter) of the cavity to reposition the electrode much closer to the AI location. As a result, a much prominent wave V of the eABR was seen at a shorter latency of 3.8 ms which is similar to cochlea with no inner ear malformations.

The above-shown wave V prominence for those stimulated contacts that are in closer proximity to the AI location, is supported by the theoretical belief that in the normal development of an inner ear during embryology, the ventral portion of the otic vesicle elongates in the ventral direction, initiating cochlear development. Therefore, the anteroinferior part of CC deformity might be programmed to differentiate to a cochlea.

Pre-curve electrode can never be positioned closer to the narrow AI location, due to the electrode's fixed size and shape, making the flexible and a straight electrode with the silicone dummy extension as a safe electrode choice for this malformation type.

4.9   Conclusion

This chapter covered the size, shape, and anatomical variations of the common cavity (CC). Majority of the CC cases what is seen clinically are not classic CC but the vestibular cavity with a complete absence if not a tiny bud-like cochlear presence. It is of importance to measure the size of the cavity from the preoperative image followed by choosing an electrode array length that matches the cavity size. A modified electrode design as proposed by Prof. Beltrame and following his modified surgical approach would ensure a safe electrode placement inside the cochlea with no chances of electrode entering the IAC. Positioning the electrode close to the anteroinferior location of the cavity is seen to evoke effective auditory sensation. With the neural elements are present along the periphery of the cavity, a pre-curved electrode with the contacts facing the inner curvature cannot be effective in the CC cases and moreover, one sized/shaped pre-curved electrode cannot offer an optimal electrode to cavity fit.

References

Beltrame MA, Bonfioli F, Frau GN. Cochlear implant in inner ear malformation: double posterior labyrinthotomy approach to common cavity. Adv Otorhinolaryngol. 2000;57:113–9.

Beltrame MA, Frau GN, Shanks M, Robinson P, Anderson I. Double posterior labyrinthotomy technique: results in three Med-El patients with common cavity. Otol Neurotol. 2005 Mar;26(2):177–82.

Beltrame MA, Birman CS, Cervera Escario J, Kassouma J, Manolidis S, Pringle MB, Robinson P, Sainz Quevedo M, Shanks M, Suckfüll M, Tomás BM. Common cavity and custom-made electrodes: speech perception and audiological performance of children with common cavity implanted with a custom-made MED-EL electrode. Int J Pediatr Otorhinolaryngol. 2013 Aug;77(8):1237–43.

Bloom JD, Rizzi MD, Germiller JA. Real-time intraoperative computed tomography to assist cochlear implant placement in the malformed inner ear. Otol Neurotol. 2009 Jan;30(1):23–6.

Cock E. A contribution to the pathology of congenital deafness. Guys Hosp Rep. 1838;7:289–307.

Dhanasingh A, Jolly C. An overview of cochlear implant electrode array designs. Hear Res. 2017 Dec; 356:93–103. https://doi.org/10.1016/j.heares.2017.10.005. Epub 2017 Oct 18. PMID: 29102129.

Graham JM, Phelps PD, Michaels L. Congenital malformations of the ear and cochlear implantation in children: review and temporal bone report of common cavity. J Laryngol Otol Suppl. 2000;25:1–14.

Kimura Y, Masuda T, Tomizawa A, Sakata H, Kaga K. A child with severe inner ear malformations with favorable hearing utilization and balance functions after wearing hearing aids. J Otol. 2017 Mar;12(1):41–6.

Manolidis S, Tonini R, Spitzer J. Endoscopically guided placement of prefabricated cochlear implant electrodes in a common cavity malformation. Int J Pediatr Otorhinolaryngol. 2006 Apr;70(4):591–6.

McElveen JT Jr, Carrasco VN, Miyamoto RT, Linthicum FH Jr. Cochlear implantation in common cavity malformations using a transmastoid labyrinthotomy approach. Laryngoscope. 1997 Aug;107(8):1032–6.

Mylanus EA, Rotteveel LJ, Leeuw RL. Congenital malformation of the inner ear and pediatric cochlear implantation. Otol Neurotol. 2004 May;25(3):308–17.

Sennaroglu L, Sarac S, Ergin T. Surgical results of cochlear implantation in malformed cochlea. Otol Neurotol. 2006 Aug;27(5):615–23.

Tucci DL, Telian SA, Zimmerman-Phillips S, Zwolen TA, Kileny PR. Cochlear implantation in patients with cochlear malformations. Arch Otolaryngol Head Neck Surg. 1995;121:833–8.

Wei X, Li Y, Fu QJ, Gong Y, Chen B, Chen J, Shi Y, Su Q, Cui D, Liu T. Slotted labyrinthotomy approach with customized electrode for patients with common cavity deformity. Laryngoscope. 2018 Feb;128(2):468–72.

Weiss NM, Langner S, Mlynski R, Roland P, Dhanasingh A. Evaluating common cavity cochlear deformities using CT images and 3D reconstruction. Laryngoscope. 2021 Feb;131(2):386–391.

Yamazaki H, Naito Y, Fujiwara K, Moroto S, Yamamoto R, Yamazaki T, Sasaki I. Electrically evoked auditory brainstem response-based evaluation of the spatial distribution of auditory neuronal tissue in common cavity deformities. Otol Neurotol. 2014 Sep;35(8):1394–402.

Yiin RS, Tang PH, Tan TY. Review of congenital inner ear abnormalities on CT temporal bone. Br J Radiol. 2011 Sep;84(1005):859–63.

Cochlear Implantation Technique for Common Cavity Deformity

5

Yongxin Li, Xingmei Wei, Jingyuan Chen, Jie Wang, Xinping Hao, and Simeng Lu

5.1 Surgical Approaches

5.1.1 The Transmastoid Facial Recess Approach

The transmastoid facial recess approach is a conventional surgical approach for CI, which includes making a posterior auricular incision, opening the mastoid process, locating the facial nerve, opening the facial recess, exposing the round window through the facial recess, and implanting electrode (Fig. 5.1). But for patients with inner ear malformations, they often accompanied with facial nerve deformity, and the incidence rate was about 14–16% (McElveen et al. 1997; Pakdaman et al. 2011), and even as high as 33–52.3% in CCD (Khan and Mikulec 2005). Therefore, for CCD, the transmastoid facial recess approach is inclined to damage the facial nerve (Molter et al. 1993). If the facial recess approach is used, facial nerve monitoring is required during the operation. In 1986, Miyamoto et al. (1986) firstly used the transmastoid facial recess approach for a CCD patient, in that report, due to the serious deformity, it was difficult to find the round window in the conventional position, so they used transmastoid facial recess cochleostomy approach (Jr and Iii 2010) to insert the electrode. When they opened the cochleostomy, profuse drainage cerebrospinal fluid (CSF) occurred, they wait until the fluid abates and then place the electrode array, and muscles should be packed around the electrodes to prevent CSF

The original version of this chapter was revised. The correction to this chapter can be found at https://doi.org/10.1007/978-981-16-8217-9_11

Y. Li · J. Chen · J. Wang · X. Hao · S. Lu · X. Wei (✉)
Department of Otorhinolaryngology Head and Neck Surgery, Beijing Tongren Hospital, Capital Medical University, Beijing, China

Key Laboratory of Otolaryngology Head and Neck Surgery (Capital Medical University), Ministry of Education, Beijing, China

Y. Li (ed.), *Cochlear Implantation for Common Cavity Deformity*, https://doi.org/10.1007/978-981-16-8217-9_5

47

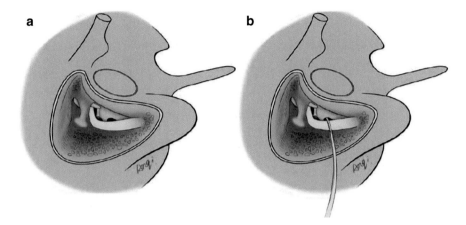

Fig. 5.1 The illustration of transmastoid facial recess approach. (**a**) Open the facial recess. (**b**) Insert the electrode through a round window

leakage. Even though, the incidence of CSF gusher during CI surgeries for CCD was as high as 38.5% (Khan and Mikulec 2005). Consequently, the surgeon should always be aware of the potential for CSF gusher and continue to explore a better way to control it.

5.1.2 Canal Wall Down Mastoidectomy Approach

Because the biggest problem of using transmastoid facial recess approach for CCD patients is to locate the cochlea and round window during surgery. In order to solve this problem, in 1995, Tucci et al. (1995) developed a canal wall down mastoidectomy approach. This approach included removing the posterior wall of external auditory canal and middle ear structures, locating the common cavity and then the labyrinthotomy was performed to implant the electrode. Finally, the external auditory canal was closed. This technique provides enough space to control the CSF gusher, but it seals the external auditory canal, which is relatively traumatic, and the operation is time consuming.

5.1.3 Transmastoid Labyrinthotomy Approach

Although some patients had been implanted electrodes through the transmastoid facial recess approach in the early years, due to the great challenge and high risk of damaging the facial nerve, the transmastoid labyrinthotomy approach was later recommended for patients with CCD (Miyamoto et al. 1986; Molter et al. 1993). This approach was firstly proposed by Molter et al. (1993) in 1993, which is also called the transmastoid external semicircular canal approach. Molter described a patient with CCD who was attempted to implant the cochlear by the transmastoid facial recess approach, but after opening facial recess, round window was atresia, and they tried to do cochleostomy, but there was soft tissue covered the location, and the facial nerve monitoring indicated the soft tissue was a bifurcated facial nerve, the position usually located lateral semicircular canal was opened and inserted the electrode array. Later, in 1997, McElveen et al. (1997) described the transmastoid labyrinthotomy in detail, and firstly used curved electrodes to avoid inserting the electrodes into the internal auditory canal (IAC). The article introduced 4 patients who underwent this approach. The beginning procedure was the same as the transmastoid facial recess approach, and the posterior auricular incision was performed and the mastoid cavity was opened. The open extent was exposure of tympanic antrum and short limb of incus, then the air cells around the common cavity were removed to fully expose the cavity, but facial recess was not opened. Then, at the position usually situated lateral semicircular canal (LSC) (Fig. 5.2a), a diamond drill is used to grind a round bony window along the long axis of the canal (parallel to the vertical segment of the facial nerve) and the common cavity was opened (Fig. 5.2b). CSF leakage may occur when the labyrinth is opened. At this moment, suction at the stoma should be avoided, and we can do sunction slowly at the mastoid cavity, and when the leak subsides with time, the electrode array can be placed. However, due to the modiolus of common cavity are absent and bone in the fundus of IAC are incomplete, the electrode is easy to be inserted into the IAC, which may stimulate the facial nerve and cause the facial twitching. To avoid the electrode into IAC, the electrode should be inserted from rear to front or use a pre-curved electrode. For example, the front end of the electrode array could be bent into a "fish hook shape," then the hook electrode is slowly implanted into the cavity and put on the wall of the cavity (Fig. 5.2c). At last, the labyrinthotomy site is closed with muscle tissues. This approach is convenient to locate the cavity, and the operation is simple and the surgery time is reduced, which can be completed within 90 min (McElveen et al. 1997), and because the insert location is far away from the facial recess, it is not susceptible to damage the facial nerve. What is more, for this approach, the cochleostomy site is located in LSC, and need not expose through the facial recess, so it is better visualized and adequate connective tissue can be packed around the electrode array to control the CSF leakage. Therefore, until 2005, a

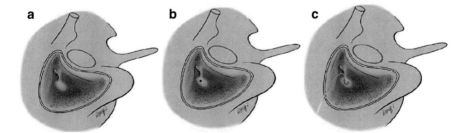

Fig. 5.2 The illustration of transmastoid labyrinthotomy approach. (**a**) The cavity's position is usually situated lateral semicircular canal; (**b**) A round bony window along the long axis of the canal (parallel to the vertical segment of the facial nerve) was ground and the common cavity was opened. (**c**) The front end of the electrode array bent into a "fish hook shape," and was slowly implanted into the cavity and put on the wall of the cavity

meta-analysis about CI surgery for CCD patients revealed that the transmastoid labyrinthotomy approach was the most frequently used surgical approach for CCD patients (Khan and Mikulec 2005).

5.1.4 Double Posterior Labyrinthotomy Approach

From the part of embryonic development, we can infer that the spiral ganglion cells are mainly located on the lateral wall of the common cavity (Graham et al. 2000). The above surgical approaches cannot ensure the electrodes are attached to the wall, which will lead to poor postoperative results or instability outcomes. To solve this problem, in 2000, Beltrame et al. (2000) modified the transmastoid labyrinthotomy as a double posterior labyrinthotomy approach and a case with Combi-40 "compressed" device was provided. Then they described the procedure detailedly in 2005 and used customized electrodes for three cases (Beltrame et al. 2005). The surgical procedure includes opening the mastoid under the microscope but not opening the facial recess, a superior labyrinthotomy was done in an area close to that where the nonampullated end of the LSC would normally be situated, and a second labyrinthotomy was done 5 mm inferior to the first (Fig. 5.3a). The two labyrinthotomy are behind the facial nerve, which reduce the probability of facial nerve injury. Then the silastic tip of the electrode array was inserted into the superior opening (Fig. 5.3b), and with the help of a hook the ending small ball was hooked and the terminal nonactive part of the electrode array was pulled out (Fig. 5.3c). Then the electrodes array was gently pushed attached to the outer sidewall of the cavity by operating the two ends of the electrode (Fig. 5.3d). The two labyrinthotomy sites were closed with muscles and connective tissue. If necessary, the packed tissues can be fixed with biological glue. This technique requires special electrodes, which are different from ordinary electrode arrays and the stimulation electrodes are placed in the middle of the electrode arrays and the end is a platinum ball (see Chap. 5 for detailed information about the electrode). This approach is easy to fix the electrode array and at the same time avoids inserting the array into the IAC. However, the disadvantage of this approach is difficult to operate and time consuming. After the electrode entered the first labyrinthotomy, it was difficult to take the electrode out from the second labyrinthotomy due to the difficulty of view in the cavity. What is more, there were two incisions needing to be filled, which may increase the possibility of CSF leakage. To solve the above disadvantage of this approach, some surgeon have proposed some methods, such as using of endoscopic to help locating the electrode (Manolidis et al. 2006), fluoroscopic microscope (Coelho et al. 2008), and real-time intraoperative CT to view the electrode (Bloom et al. 2009). In 2006, Manolidis et al. (2006) reported a method of using an endoscope to achieve accurate positioning of electrodes under direct vision (Fig. 5.4). The detailed procedures were creating a third opening in the labyrinth, implanting an endoscope with a diameter of 2 mm which helps look directly into the structures inside the common cavity, and placing the customized electrodes accurately. However, the disadvantage of this method is that an

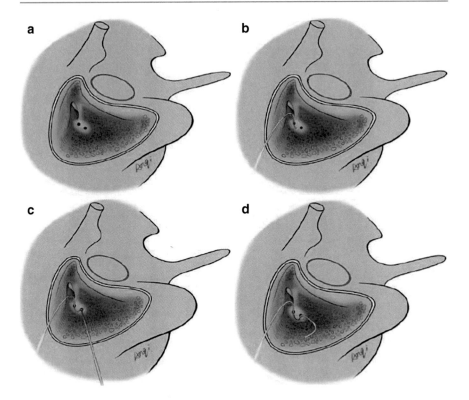

Fig. 5.3 The double posterior labyrinthotomy approach. (**a**) Two labyrinthotomy was done in an area where the lateral semicircular canal is normally situated. (**b**) The electrode array was inserted into the superior opening. (**c**) A hook was used to pull the electrode array out. (**d**) The electrode array was gently pushed attached to the outer sidewall of the cavity by operating the two ends of the electrode

additional opening is added and the entire surgical process is more complicated. Fishman et al. (2003) and Coelho et al. (2008) also used a fluoroscopy microscope to locate the electrodes, which can clearly see the location of the common cavity and avoid inserting the electrode into IAC (Fig. 5.5). In addition, Bloom et al. (2009) also proposed the use of intraoperative real-time CT positioning to help achieve electrode locating during CI surgery for CCD (Fig. 5.6). However, all of the above methods require expensive and complicated equipments, and the latter two even let the surgeon and patients under radiation during the operation, which limits their application.

5.1.5 Single-Slit Labyrinthotomy

Due to the difficult operation of double posterior labyrinthotomy, the two openings are more traumatic, and CSF leakage is more likely to occur. In 2010, Sennaroglu

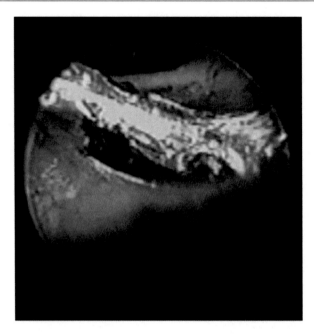

Fig. 5.4 Endoscopic view of the common cavity during electrode positioning (reproduced with permission from Manolidis et al. 2006)

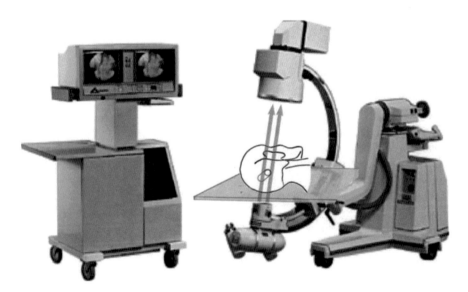

Fig. 5.5 The C-arm of the mobile fluoroscopy unit (reproduced with permission from Coelho et al. 2008)

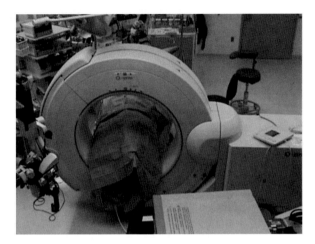

Fig. 5.6 View of the O-Arm and room setup (reproduced with permission from Bloom et al. 2009)

(2010) mentioned in his review about inner ear malformation classification and CI surgery that J Graham recommended the single-slit labyrinthotomy, but it was not described in detail in that article. In 2011, Wang et al. (Bin et al. 2011) first described single-slit labyrinthotomy in a Chinese article. They made a 1.0 mm × 3.0 mm labyrinthotomy in the position of LSC, and put the electrode in the cavity in a "U" shape, and a little muscle was used to close the labyrinthotomy site. In 2013, Beltrame et al. (2013) introduced the single-slit cochleostomy approach in detail with the use of customized electrodes. The procedures include an incision behind the auricle, opening the mastoid, but not opening the facial recess, making a long labyrinthotomy at the same position as the double posterior labyrinthotomy, where the LSC was usually located, and the size was about 1.0 mm × 4.0 mm. The customized electrode was curved pushed into the cavity. This approach does not require the electrode to be hooked out, which is convenient, and the surgery can be completed quickly. However, Beltrame et al. considered that compared the double posterior labyrinthotomy with a single-slit labyrinthotomy, the former has a smaller opening and a lower incidence of CSF leakage. In order to solve the problem of CSF leakage, in 2015, Xia et al. (2015) modified this approach. And the improvement was that after implanting electrodes in the cochleostomy, the muscle and fascia were fully packed in the cochleostomy, which can fill the cavity to avoid postoperative CSF leakage, and can force the electrodes attached to the wall. However, this report did not use customized electrodes, and for ordinary electrodes, the electrodes are located at the end of arrays, it is not convenient to be fixed in the common cavity and is not good for preventing electrodes from entering into IAC. In 2018, Wei et al. (2018) reported the modified single-slit labyrinthotomy with custom electrodes, which was used for 7 patients of CCD, and named it as transmastoid slotted labyrinthotomy approach with customized electrode. The surgical procedure includes making a "C" shaped incision about 3 cm long, 5 mm above the mastoid tip, and 5–10 mm posterior the auricle. The bone cortex of the mastoid surface was completely chiseled off. After the common cavity bone wall was exposed by traditional mastoidectomy, a single-slit labyrinthotomy was made at the position of LSC, which was about 1.0 mm × 4.0 mm and parallel to facial nerve (Fig. 5.7a). Be careful to protect the facial nerve during the labyrinthotomy. After the labyrinthotomy, lymph fluid may flow out from the common cavity. When the lymphatic fluid overflows slowly or stops, the electrodes were inserted (Fig. 5.7b). The electrodes are all customized electrodes. When inserting, the electrodes were bent into a "U" shape, and slowly placed into the cavity using microscopic instruments (Fig. 5.7c). Then muscle or fascia were used to fill the common cavity, which made the electrodes closely contact the cavity wall, and the muscle also can seal the cochleostomy site and prevent CSF leakage (Fig. 5.7d). Currently, our team has used this approach for more than 40 CCD patients. All the patients had no postoperative CSF leakage and facial nerve injury. In the same year, Józef et al. (2018) used the same approach for five CCD patients, and they did a modification and emphasized the cochleostomy shape should be like a "banana" to prevent the electrode slippage, and they named it as "banana cochleostomy approach" (Fig. 5.8). In our cases, the

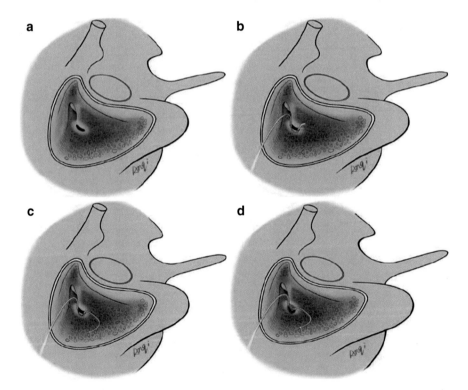

Fig. 5.7 The illustration of the transmastoid slotted labyrinthotomy approach. (**a**) A single-slit labyrinthotomy of 1.0 mm × 4.0 mm was made at the position of lateral semicircular canal; (**b**) Insert the electrode; (**c**) The electrodes were bent into a "U" shape, and slowly placed into the cavity using microscopic instruments; (**d**) The cavity was packed with muscle or fascia, and forced the electrodes to the cavity wall

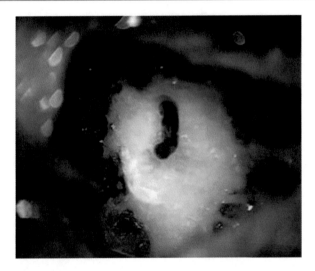

Fig. 5.8 Opening the cavity and creating the "banana cochleostomy" (reproduced with permission from Józef et al. 2018)

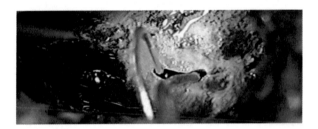

Fig. 5.9 The single-slit labyrinthotomy with looped electrode

cochleostomy shapes are also cambered (Fig. 5.9), actually, the size, shape, and accurate location of labyrinthotomy should be produced according to the specific patient's characteristics. In 2021, Hu et al. (2020) proposed a rounded insertion technique (RIT) for CCD and cochlear hypoplasia patients, which is actually a modification of single-slit labyrinthotomy. RIT emphasized inserting the electrode array looped in the middle region and the tip of the electrode array was fixed to one side of the labyrinthotomy but away from the cavity, whereas the other end was inserted in a manner to ensure the electrode array contacted the wall and not into the IAC (Fig. 5.10). RIT can keep the electrode lying against the cavity during surgery, and donut-shaped facia was sealed in the opening, but it did not use muscle filling in the cavity to keep the electrode fixed and lacked long-time follow-up images. What is more, from the surgical images in Fig. 5.11 we can notice that the top and tip electrodes were closed to each other at the labyrinthotomy site, which may cause resistance interference between electrodes and long time programing follow up should be recorded.

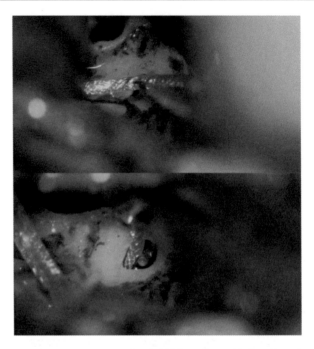

Fig. 5.10 The electrode array was looped in the middle region and inserted into the opening of the common cavity (reproduced with permission from Hu et al. 2020)

5.2 Intraoperative Monitoring for CCD

5.2.1 Electrically Evoked Auditory Brainstem Responses

Since patients with CCD are often accompanied by cochlear nerve deficiency, if the patient has no clear residual hearing before surgery, the postoperative outcome is uncertain. During the surgery, it is necessary to do intraoperative audiology monitoring to determine the function of the entire auditory pathway. Electrically evoked auditory brainstem responses (EABR) is the most commonly used electrophysiological test to evaluate the auditory system during CI. Bin et al. (2013) reported that EABR test was performed after the common cavity was opened during surgery. If a meaningful waveform can be identified, a cochlear implant will be performed; if it cannot be identified, the operation will be terminated. He studied 16 CCD patients with no objective residual hearing before surgery, all of them induced V waves during surgery, and they can get hearing after surgery. They also found that the EABR test for CCD patients required greater stimulation levels which was significantly higher than that of normal patients, to elicit meaningful waves. Other studies also found that EABR in CCD patients requires a larger pulse width, and the wave shapes were worse than that in patients without deformities (Papsin 2005). In 2014, Yamazaki et al. (2014) also tried to reveal the distribution of auditory neuronal in

Fig. 5.11 The EABR
waves in a patient
with CCD

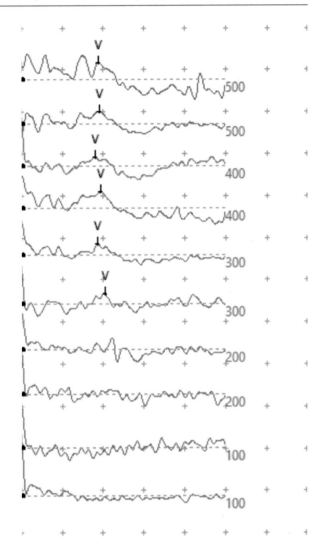

the common cavity through intraoperative EABR monitoring. The tests were introduced by opening the common cavity through labyrinthotomy, and EABR is tested
after implanting electrodes. A total of 5 patients were tested, and the results were
that the anteroinferior wall of the common cavity can all elicit evoked V waves, and
the incubation period is similar to that of patients with normal cochlea, so they concluded that more auditory neuronal elements are distributed to the anteroinferior
part of CCD. This research instructed surgeon to place electrodes to the anteroinferior part of the cavity for CCD patients. To confirm more auditory neurons are
located in the bottom of common cavity (near IAC), we performed preoperative
EABR with MEDEL clinical system during surgery. After the cavity was open, a
PromStim electrode was placed at the bottom of the common cavity to record the

EABR and the wave was elicited (Fig. 5.11). However, before the cavity was open, the electrode on the labyrinth cannot elicit waves. The best position and angle of electrode array in common cavity need further research and EABR may be a useful technique.

5.2.2   Auditory Nerve Response Telemetry

In addition, the auditory nerve response telemetry (ART) technology can monitor the patient's electrically evoked compound action potentials (eCAP) to determine the function of peripheral auditory pathway. We performed impedance tests and ART in 14 CCD patients during CI surgery,13 patients were MEDEL, and the other one was Cochlear implants. After the connection of receiver and intracorporeal device is completed, the impedances of each electrode were tested first to confirm the integrity of the implant, and then, using MAESTRO System Software or the Custom Sound EP to measure the ART according to the different implants. Generally, we tested all electrodes unless some of them had high impedance. For MEDEL implants, the electrical pulse signal is commanded by the Maestro software, and the cochlear implant electrodes are stimulated by a common ground single electrode mode. The maximum stimulus intensity is 1000 cu, the minimum is 100 cu, and the decreasing step distance is 225 cu. The eCAP waves and amplitudes are recorded automatically and identified by experienced audiologists (Fig. 5.12). Our results showed that the total positive rate of ART was 8.0% (14/177), ART was elicited in 3/14 patients, which was much lower than non-malformation patients (Shi et al. 2019). The results concluded that the intraoperative ART positive rate of CCD patients is lower than that of normal cochlea patients, which may be related to the fewer CCD spiral ganglia and auditory nerve fibers. Therefore, some researchers suggested that for such patients with severe inner ear malformations and cochlear nerve deficiency, the eCAP test requires a larger amount of stimulation to elicit a response (Buchman et al. 2011; He et al. 2018), for example, by increasing the pulse phase duration. Moreover, the electrode response amplitude is different from that of

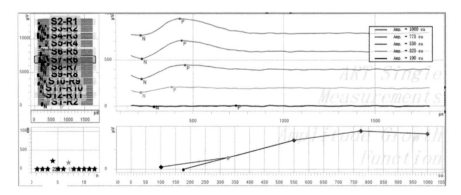

Fig. 5.12   The intraoperative ART test picture of testing 12 electrodes

normal patients, which has a gradual upward trend from the bottom of the cochlea to the top of the cochlea. It may be due to the small sample and low positive rate, the amplitude varied pattern has not been found. However, the study also found that for children whose ART were negative, the auditory response could still be obtained after surgery, which can conclude that ART can only be used as an auxiliary judgement for prognosis. The average impedance of endocochlear electrodes was below 5 kΩ, which has no significant difference with normal cochlea (Shi et al. 2019). It may be because that the impedance of the electrode has no significant relationship with the deformity of the cochlea and its main influencing factors are the amount of lymph around the electrode, the proliferation of inflammatory fibrous tissue in the cochlea, and the design of the implanted electrode (Franck and Shah 2004).

In addition, we also found the positive eCAP of our patients mainly located in the middle electrodes, such as electrodes 6 and 7, which may be because these patients all used slotted labyrinthotomy approach and implanted the customized electrodes, and the electrodes were placed in U shape. The middle electrodes were located at the bottom of the common cavity. According to the first chapter, we know that the closer to the bottom of the common cavity (near IAC), the more spiral ganglion cells are distributed. The higher eCAP positive rate in this part may be related to more auditory cells in this part. The results above may provide a research foundation for our future surgical methods development and electrode design for CCD patients.

EABR and eCAP tests both have advantages and disadvantages, and their functions and reflected auditory pathways are different. The former reflects the function of the entire auditory pathway, including the advanced auditory center; the latter mainly reflects the function of the peripheral auditory pathway. The advantage of the former is that the incubation period is longer than that of the latter, however it is likely to be concealed by stimulus interference. And the positive rate for patients with inner ear malformations is much higher using EABR, which can reflect the activities of higher-level central centers. The eCAP has the advantages of simple equipment, fast test speed, strong recording signal, simple procedure, and not being affected by mental state, muscles, and anesthesia. The combination of the two methods can better reflect and monitor the activities of the auditory function during operation in real time.

5.3   Case Reports

We will share some of CCD's special cases below. From these cases, we will share our experiences on surgery sides selected strategies and surgical techniques in some special conditions.

5.3.1   Case 1

A 2-year-old boy, with bilateral CCD, the first one underwent sequential bilateral CI surgery. His preoperative CT displayed bilateral CCD (Fig. 5.13a), but the left showed some soft tissue density shadow in the middle ear cavity. According to our experiences, CSF leakage in the left side should be considered. So we choose the left side to do surgery first. His left ear implanted cochlear by TSLA using customized electrode (MED-EL) in April 2018. During surgery, there was certainly CSF leakage and we did CI and leakage repair at the same time. After 7 months, his right side was implanted CI (Fig. 5.13b–d). The postoperative CT showed the electrodes of both sides were in the cavity and located well (Fig. 5.13e, f). Three years after surgery, his CAP, SIR, IT-MAIS, and MUSS scores were 7, 5, 40, and 40, respectively. The closed two-syllable speech recognition rate in a quiet environment was 95%, and the short sentence recognition rate was 100%.

5.3.2 Case 2

A 10-month-old girl, with bilateral CCD (Fig. 5.14a, b) and cochlear nerve deficiency (CND) (Fig. 5.14c, d) underwent CI surgery in her right ear by TSLA using CI24RE(ST) electrode (Cochlear, Australia) in December 2019. From oblique

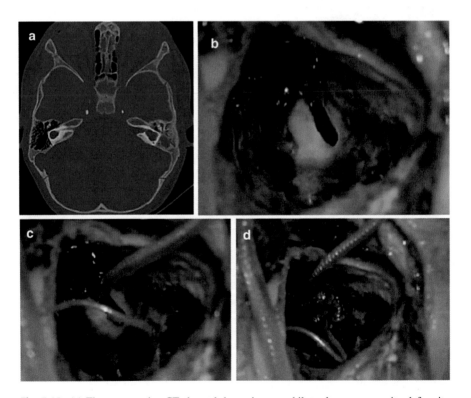

Fig. 5.13 (**a**) The preoperative CT showed the patient was bilateral common cavity deformity (**b–d**). (**b**) The cavity was opened; (**c**) The electrode array was implanted in the cavity; (**d**) The cavity was filled with muscle. (**e, f**) The axial (**e**) and coronal (**f**) position of postoperative CT

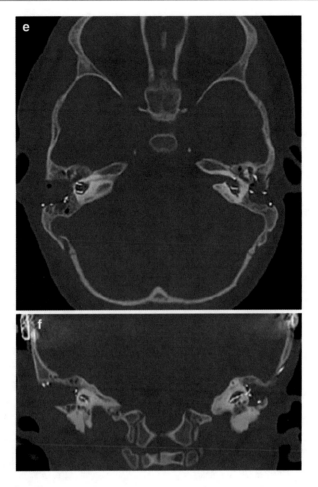

Fig. 5.13 (continued)

sagittal position of the inner ear MRI, there was two obscure nerve bundle in the IAC of her right side, and an obvious nerve bundle in her left side. And there was no residual hearing observed from her preoperative auditory examinations. We choose her right side for CI. During surgery, when opening the cavity, we found there was cerebrospinal fluid (CSF) leakage, and we implanted the electrode in the cavity and filled the cavity with lots of muscle to stop the CSF leakage and fixed the electrode array (Fig. 5.14e, f, g). We also observed that neural reflection telemetry (NRT) could be recorded during surgery (Fig. 5.14h). Her postoperative CT showed the electrodes were all in the cavity (Fig. 5.14i, j). The patient's postoperative performance was good. Eighteen months after surgery, her CAP, SIR, IT-MAIS, and MUSS scores were 5, 2, 24, and 9, respectively. Then the patient received left CI in May 2021 and became a bilateral CI user. Three months later, her closed two-syllable speech recognition rate in a quiet environment was 66.7%. This case

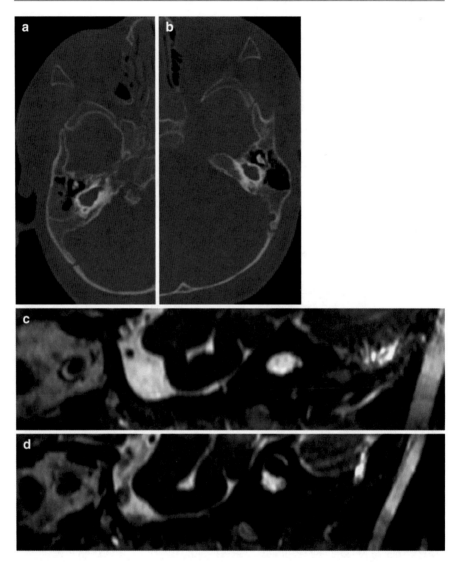

Fig. 5.14 (a) Temporal bone CT of the right side. (b) Temporal bone CT of left side. (c) The right ear's oblique sagittal position of MRI showed there were two blurry nerve bundles in the internal auditory canal (IAC). (d) The left ear's oblique sagittal position of MRI showed there were no obvious nerve bundles. (e) The cavity was opened; (f) The electrode array was implanted in the cavity; (g) The cavity was filled with muscle. (h) The neural reflection telemetry elicited waves. (i, j) The postoperative temporal bone showed the electrode was in the cavity

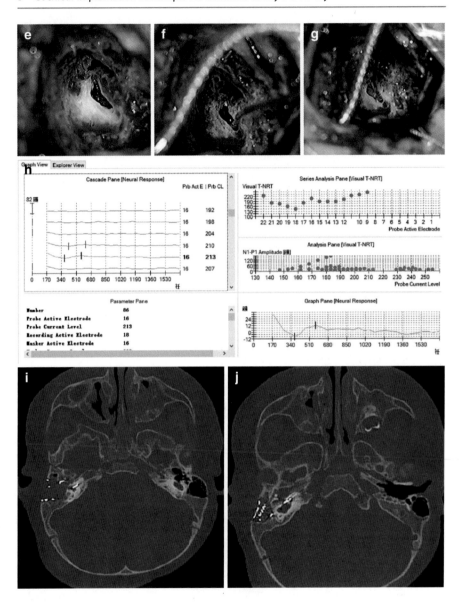

Fig. 5.14 (continued)

indicated us CCD may accompany by CSF leakage and TSLA approach can control the leakage and postoperative performance is not affected.

5.3.3 Case 3

A 2-year-old girl, with bilateral CCD, underwent CI surgery in her left ear by TSLA using customized electrode (MED-EL) in October 2019. On the CT scan (Fig. 5.15a), there is a bone island in the cavity. During surgery, when opening the cavity, a bone island appeared, then we drilled the bone island and implanted the electrode and filled the cavity with muscle (Fig. 5.15b–f). And postoperative CT showed the electrode array was located in the cavity and electrodes were closed to the cavity wall (Fig. 5.15g, h). Eighteen months after surgery, her CAP, SIR, IT-MAIS, and MUSS scores were 5, 2, 37, and 2, respectively. This case indicated us the embryonic development of CCD stopped at different times, and sometimes some structures of vestibule were formed, such as semicircular canal and bone island. In order to implant the electrode, some structures could be removed.

5.3.4 Case 4

A 1 years and 7 months old boy, with bilateral CCD (Fig. 5.16a) and CND (Fig. 5.16b,c) underwent CI surgery in his right ear by TSLA using customized electrode (MED-EL) in July 2019. His preoperative inner ear MRI showed that the nerve bundle in his right side was 2, but on the left side there was no nerve bundle.

Fig. 5.15 (a) The preoperative CT showed the patient was bilateral common cavity deformity. (b) The cavity was opened, and there was a bone island in the cavity. (c) The bone island was drilled. (d) After the bone island drilled, there was a big cavity. (e) The electrode array was implanted in the cavity. (f) The cavity was filled with muscle. (g, h) The postoperative CT scan showed the electrode array was located well in the cavity

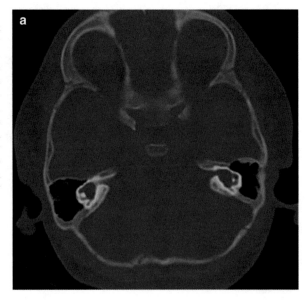

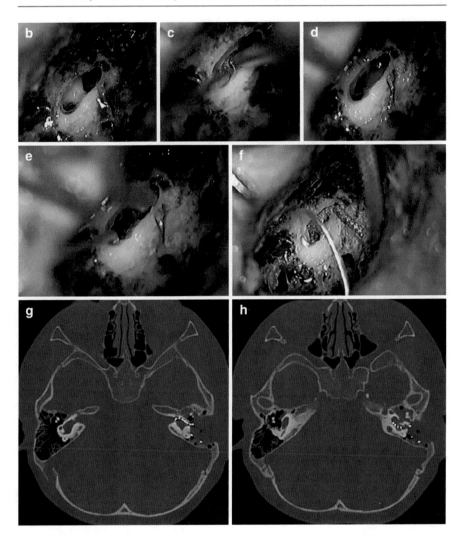

Fig. 5.15 (continued)

We choosed the right side for CI. The surgical procedure was shown in Fig. 5.16d–g. The patient's NRT during surgery also can be observed (Fig. 5.12). The postoperative CT showed the electrode's position was good (Fig. 5.16h). His CAP, SIR, IT-MAIS, and MUSS scores 2 years after surgery were 5, 3, 39, and 15, respectively, which were better among the CND patients and the closed two-syllable speech recognition rate in a quiet environment was 63.3%.

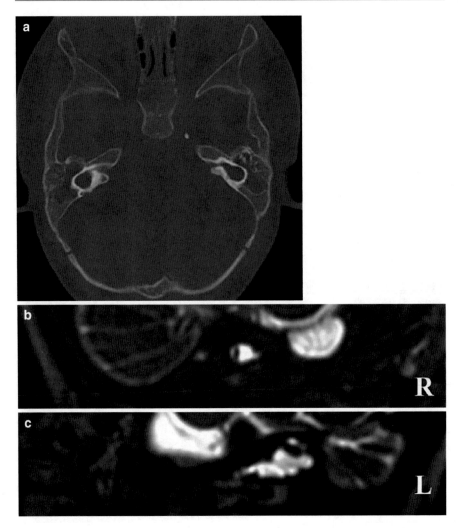

Fig. 5.16 (**a**) The preoperative CT showed the patient was bilateral common cavity deformity (**b**, **c**). (**b**). The right ear's oblique sagittal position of MRI showed there was one nerve bundle in the internal auditory canal (IAC). (**c**) The left ear's oblique sagittal position of MRI showed there was no obvious nerve bundle (**d–g**). (**d**) The membrane of labyrinth was exposed; (**e**) The cavity was opened; (**f**) The electrode array was implanted in the cavity; (**g**) The cavity was filled with muscle; (**h**) The postoperative CT scan showed the electrode array was located well in the cavity

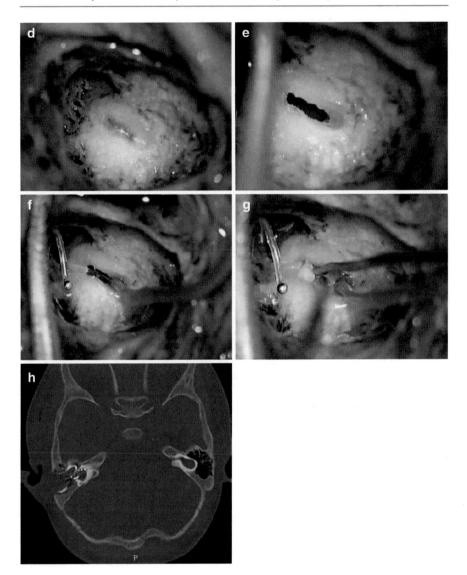

Fig. 5.16 (continued)

5.4 Conclusion

CCD patients have poor residual hearing, and CI surgery is more difficult than normal patients. However, through continuous exploration, a safe, fast, and effective electrode implantation can be achieved by using a suitable approach. At present, the single-slit labyrinthotomy approach with customized electrodes is considered to be a more suitable surgical method. The positive rate for CCD patients of intraoperative electrophysiological tests is lower than that of normal patients. The use of intraoperative nerve detection technology to guide surgery needs further exploration. With the development of surgical techniques, perioperative complications such as CSF gusher, facial nerve stimulation, and electrode displacement rarely happen. CI surgery for CCD is safe.

Acknowledgement We thank Anqi Zhao from Beijing Tongren Hospital for drawing the surgical schematic diagrams of Figs. 5.1, 5.2, 5.3, and 5.7.

References

Beltrame MA, Bonfioli F, et al. Cochlear implant in inner ear malformation: double posterior labyrinthotomy approach to common cavity. Adv Otorhinolaryngol. 2000;57:113.

Beltrame MA, Frau GN, et al. Double posterior labyrinthotomy technique: results in three med-El patients with common cavity. Otol Neurotol. 2005;26(2):177–82.

Beltrame MA, Birman CS, et al. Common cavity and custom-made electrodes: speech perception and audiological performance of children with common cavity implanted with a custom-made MED-EL electrode. Int J Pediatr Otorhinolaryngol. 2013;77(8):1237–43.

Bin W, Chaogang W, et al. The assessment of cochlear implantation assisted by EABR in patients with common cavity deformity. J Clin Otorhinolaryngol Head Neck Surg. 2011;25(10):436–40.

Bin W, Keli C, et al. Evaluation of the intro-operative EABR characteristics and the rehabilitation effects in patients with common cavity deformity. Chinese Arch Otolaryngol Head Neck Surg. 2013;20(5):239–43.

Bloom JD, Rizzi MD, et al. Real-time intraoperative computed tomography to assist cochlear implant placement in the malformed inner ear. Otol Neurotol. 2009;30(1):23–6.

Buchman CA, Teagle HFB, et al. Cochlear implantation in children with labyrinthine anomalies and cochlear nerve deficiency: implications for auditory brainstem implantation. Laryngoscope. 2011;121(9):1979–88.

Coelho DH, Waltzman SB, et al. Implanting common cavity malformations using intraoperative fluoroscopy. Otol Neurotol. 2008;29(7):914–9.

Fishman AJ, Roland JT, et al. Fluoroscopically assisted cochlear implantation. Otol Neurotol. 2003;24(6):882.

Franck KH, Shah UK. Averaged electrode voltage testing to diagnose an unusual Cochlear implant internal device failure. J Am Acad Audiol. 2004;15(9):643–8.

Graham JM, Phelps PD, et al. Congenital malformations of the ear and cochlear implantation in children: review and temporal bone report of common cavity. J Laryngol Otol Suppl. 2000;25(S25):1–14.

He S, Shahsavarani BS, et al. Responsiveness of the electrically stimulated Cochlear nerve in children with Cochlear nerve deficiency. Ear & Hearing. 2018;1

Hu H, Chen WK, et al. Rounded insertion technique for Cochlear implantation surgery to treat cystic inner ear malformation. Laryngoscope. 2020;130(9):2229–33.

Józef M, Egwin VDH, et al. Application of "banana cochleostomy" and looped electrode insertion for cochlear implantation in children with common cavity malformation and cystic forms of cochlear hypoplasia. Int J Pediatr Otorhinolaryngol. 2018;112:16–23.

Jr ME, Iii CDC. Cochlear implantation in the congenitally malformed ear. Otolaryngol Head Neck Surg. 2010;21(4):243–7.

Khan AM, Mikulec A. Cochlear implantation in the common cavity deformity. Otolaryngol Head Neck Surg. 2005;133(2):P234–4.

Manolidis S, Tonini R, et al. Endoscopically guided placement of prefabricated cochlear implant electrodes in a common cavity malformation. Int J Pediatr Otorhinolaryngol. 2006;70(4):591–6.

McElveen JT Jr, Carrasco VN, Miyamoto RT, Linthicum FH Jr. Cochlear implantation in common cavity malformations using a transmastoid labyrinthotomy approach. Laryngoscope. 1997;107(8):1032–6.

Miyamoto RT, Robbins AJ, et al. Cochlear implantation in the Mondini inner ear malformation. Am J Otol. 1986;7(4):258.

Molter DW, Pate BR, et al. Cochlear implantation in the congenitally malformed ear. Otolaryngol Head Neck Surg. 1993;108(2):174–7.

Pakdaman MN, Herrmann BS, et al. Cochlear implantation in children with anomalous Cochleovestibular anatomy. Otolaryngol Head Neck Surg. 2011;146(2):180–90.

Papsin B. Cochlear implantation in children with anomalous chochleovestibular anatomy. Laryngoscope. 2005;115

Sennaroglu L. Cochlear implantation in inner ear malformations--a review article. Cochlear Implants Int. 2010;11(1):4–41.

Shi, Y., B. Chen, et al. Transmastoidslotted labyrinthotomy approach cochlear implantation with customized electrode for patients with common cavity deformity. 2019

Tucci DL, Telian SA, et al. Cochlear implantation in patients with Cochlear malformations. Arch Otolaryngol Head Neck Surg. 1995;121(8):833–8.

Wei X, Li Y, et al. Slotted labyrinthotomy approach with customized electrode for patients with common cavity deformity. Laryngoscope. 2018;128(2)

Xia J, Wang W, et al. Cochlear implantation in 21 patients with common cavity malformation. Acta Otolaryngol. 2015;135(5):459–65.

Yamazaki H, Naito Y, et al. Electrically evoked auditory brainstem response-based evaluation of the spatial distribution of auditory neuronal tissue in common cavity deformities. Otol Neurotol. 2014;35(8):1394–402.

Cochlear Implantation Complications and the Management for Common Cavity Deformity

Biao Chen, Xingmei Wei, Jingyuan Chen, and Yongxin Li

Cochlear implantation (CI) is the most effective treatment for many profound hearing loss patients. Although it is a relatively safe surgical procedure, revision surgeries are sometimes necessary because of the complication. Some studies have reported the rate of surgical complications, including major complications and minor complication, were 4–19.9% (Cohen et al., 1988; Masterson et al., 2012; Farinetti et al., 2014). Cohen et al. categorized the complications as major and minor firstly, and distinguished the complications from whether threatened life (Cohen et al., 1988). Major complication means the revision surgery was necessary and minor complication means it could be resolved spontaneously or with minimal treatment (Cohen et al., 1988). The most common complications after CI surgery for CCD include CSF gusher, meningitis, facial never injury, facial nerve stimulation, electrode displacement, and vestibular stimulation. We will discuss them below.

6.1 Cerebrospinal Fluid Gusher

Gusher is one type of cerebrospinal fluid (CSF) leakage. In 1994, Phelps et al. (1994) divided CSF leakage into two types: oozing and gusher (Phelps et al. 1994). A gentle flow of clear fluid is called "oozing" and a profuse flow is termed as "gusher." Different from "oozing," the CSF gusher always lasts longer because of a

B. Chen (✉) · X. Wei · J. Chen · Y. Li
Department of Otorhinolaryngology Head and Neck Surgery, Beijing Tongren Hospital, Capital Medical University, Beijing, China

Key Laboratory of Otolaryngology Head and Neck Surgery (Capital Medical University), Ministry of Education, Beijing, China

© The Author(s), under exclusive license to Springer Nature Singapore Pte Ltd. 2022
Y. Li (ed.), *Cochlear Implantation for Common Cavity Deformity*,
https://doi.org/10.1007/978-981-16-8217-9_6

bigger defect (Sennaroglu 2010). Gusher is common during CI surgery for inner ear malformation, such as CCD, incomplete partition type I (IP-I), incomplete partition type II (IP-II), incomplete partition type III (IP-III), and enlarged vestibular aqueduct (EVA). Generally, the CSF gusher occurred because of variable size defects between the malformed inner ear and internal auditory canal (IAC) and high-resolution computerized tomography (HRCT), and magnetic resonance imaging (MRI) could demonstrate the defect. But not all patients with a defect between inner ear and IAC occurred CSF leakage during CI surgery (Fishman et al. 2003; Mylanus et al. 2004, 2006; Beltrame et al. 2005). The reason for CSF leakage is undefined completely, fiber stripe between IAC and cochlea may play an important role. For severe inner ear malformation (IEM), such as CCD, IP-I, or IP-III, there is a wide communication between the malformed inner ear and the subarachnoid space, so during cochleostomy in these patients, the CSF gusher usually lasts for 10–20 min (Sennaroglu et al. 2006; Incesulu et al. 2008).

The first report of CSF gusher during CI surgery was by Miyamoto et al. (1986), and it occurred in a patient with CCD. The incidences of CSF gusher in different inner ear malformation were variable, and it was relatively high in CCD patients. Hoffman et al. (1997) reported 21 of 50 patients with inner ear malformation occurred CSF leakage during surgery, among which 50% were CCD. Papsin (2005) reviewed 103 patients with anomalous cochleovestibular anatomy, 7 occurred CSF gusher, among which 3 were CCD.

Perioperative management of CSF leakage is very important because if it fails, there is a risk of permanent CSF leakage with a potential risk of meningitis. Now with the improvement of surgical technique and experience, such as reduced surgical time, use of soft tissue around the cochleostomy, custom made electrode with "cork" stopper, and timely postoperative treatments, the gusher during CCD patients' CI surgery can be controlled, and if it occurred, it was mainly oozing, which will not cause a severe consequence. Then the strategies to reduce CSF gusher will be described as follows.

6.1.1   Electrode Insertion Time

CFS gusher increases the surgical difficulty, mainly because the occlusion of the surgical field is difficult for electrode implantation and increases the difficulty of plugging the leakage (Graham et al. 2000). Therefore, surgeons usually need to wait until the gusher slows down before performing electrode insertion (Fig. 6.1) and the waiting time is usually 10–20 min, which is an appropriate time to insert the electrode and pack soft tissue.

6.1.2   Use of Soft Tissue

Application of soft tissue is very important in cases of gusher because sufficient soft tissue can prevent the recurrence of CSF leakage (Fig. 6.2). In addition, soft tissue is also conducive to the electrode fixation in CCD and packing around the electrode should be firm. However, sometimes CSF leakage may recur several months after the surgery. A case reported by Hoffman et al. (1997) described

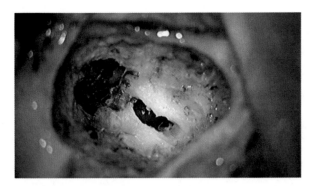

Fig. 6.1 The gusher slows down before electrode insertion

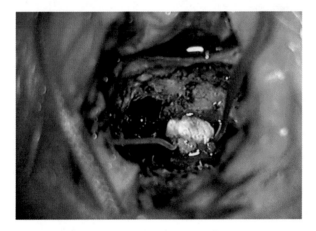

Fig. 6.2 The use of soft tissue to prevent cerebrospinal fluid gusher in common cavity deformity

partial extrusion of the electrode and accompanied with gusher in 5 months after the initial surgery (Hoffman et al. 1997). Luntz et al. (1997) also described a patient who had a slowly progressive extrusion of electrode array and three electrodes extracochlear, in the end, the patient underwent revised surgery (Luntz et al. 1997). For CCD, the size of cochleostomy is relatively big (Wei et al. 2018), so the risk of electrode extrusion and gusher increases. Therefore, fixation of the electrode is especially important in patients where there is a risk of profuse CSF gusher, since extrusion of the electrode from the cochlea can pull the sealed tissue out of the cochleostomy.

6.1.3   Custom Made Electrode with "Cork" Stopper

The first report of "cork" stopper was by Levent et al. in 2014, which was produced by Med-El company which aims to stop CSF leakage (Sennaroglu et al. 2014) (Fig. 6.3). The special electrode has a cork-like stopper instead of the usual silicon ring at the proximal end of the intracochlear electrode to prevent CSF leakage after insertion. When combined with a piece of fascia around the "cork" stopper, the sealed function will be better (Fig. 6.4). In our center, thirteen inner ear

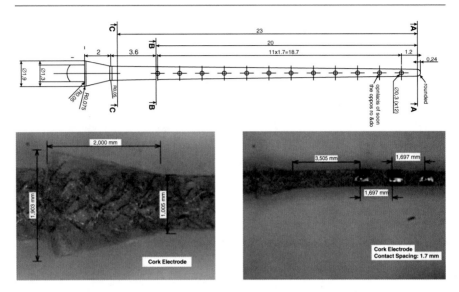

Fig. 6.3 The pictures of standard cork electrode (reproduced with permission from Sennaroglu et al. 2014)

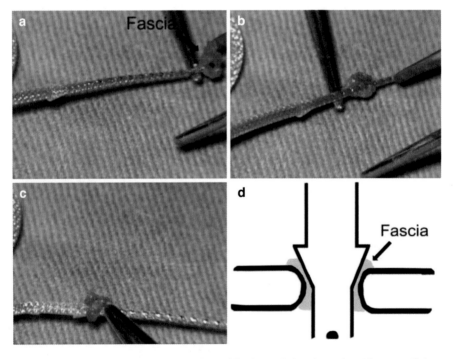

Fig. 6.4 The "cork" electrode with a tiny piece of fascia. (**a**) A tiny piece of muscle was made into a circle and put around the electrode; (**b**) pull the muscle up along the electrode; (**c**) the muscle was placed in the "cork" position; (**d**) diagram of the cochleostomy with"cork" electrode (reproduced with permission from Sennaroglu et al. 2014)

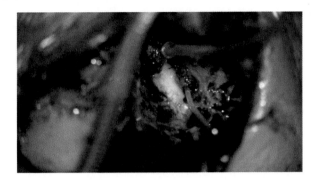

Fig. 6.5 The custom-made electrodes with "cork" stopper in CCD patients

malformations patients with CSF gusher were resolved with this new electrode. Unlike Levent, the authors of this book used custom-made electrodes with "cork" stopper by transmastoid slotted labyrinthotomy approach (TSLA) to handle CSF gusher in CCD patients (Wei et al. 2018) (Fig. 6.5).

6.1.4 Postoperative Treatment

For patients with CSF gushers during CI surgery, head elevation and bed rest for 48 h can decrease postoperative CSF leakage. In addition, acetazolamide can be used to decrease CSF production (Arimappamagan et al. 2019). The use of mannitol during surgery can reduce the intracranial pressure to make electrodes insertion easier and help seal the cochleostomy completely (Kim et al. 2006). If some patients develop rhinorrhea after surgery, continuous lumbar drainage should be performed to reduce the pressure of CSF and the CSF will be drained by the drainage tube and CSF pressure around the cochleostomy will be lower, and it is easier for the leakage site to heal (Tucci et al. 1995).

6.2 Facial Nerve Injury

Facial nerve is one of the most important structures in the temporal bone. The route of facial nerve is intricate and sometimes exhibits varied or malformed, which increases the surgical difficulty (Mandour et al. 2021). Because the facial nerve canal develops from the primordial otic capsule and Reichert's cartilage, the abnormal development of the temporal bony structures may affect the facial nerve's route. So, the patient with IEM may be accompanied by facial nerve route anomaly, (Romo and Curtin 2001; Sennaroglu and Tahir 2020), and according to researches' reports, the rate of abnormal facial nerve in IEM reached 14–16% (McElveen et al. 1997; Papsin 2005). For CCD patients, the abnormal rate of facial nerve was as high as

33% to 52.35 (Khan and Mikulec 2005), and the abnormal anatomy mainly occurred in intrapetrous part of the facial nerve and the malformed facial nerve often runs anterolaterally and is closed to the common cavity (Buchman et al. 2004). Therefore, the risk of facial nerve injury increases during CI surgery in CCD. Accurate imaging, secure planning of the surgical approach, and perioperative facial nerve monitoring are crucial to avoid this complication. For example, to avoid facial nerve injury, labyrinthotomy approaches were proposed (McElveen et al. 1997; Wei et al. 2018).

6.3 Facial Nerve Stimulation

Due to the high incidence of aberrant facial nerve in CCD (McElveen et al. 1997), stimulation is another common complication after CI surgery for CCD patients. For example, Ahmad (Ahmad and Lokman 2005) reported one CCD occurred facial nerve stimulation one and half a year after surgery because of electrode displacement. Luntz et al. reported 2 of 10 CCD patients occurred facial nerve stimulation. Because the nerve location in the cavity of CCD is different with normal cochlea, and an aberrant course of the facial nerve or a close relation between facial nerve and cochlea in the IAC may exist, the electrode may stimulate the facial nerve when activating the cochlear nerve. During the programing procedure in our center, there were some patients who also suffered from facial nerve stimulation, and by inactivating some electrodes or decreasing the stimulation current the problem could be solved. Sometimes, for severe facial nerve stimulation, a revision surgery is necessary (Lassig et al. 2005).

6.4 Electrode Displacement

The size and shape of the cavity of each CCD patient are different, and the volume of cavity varies from about 52 to 233 mm^3 (Dhanasingh et al. 2019; Weiss et al. 2021). Literature found the Corti organs in CCD patients located in peripheral sites of the cavity (Zheng et al. 2002). To obtain good auditory responses, as many as electrodes stimulate the auditory neural in the common cavity is necessary (Kaga et al. 2020). But the auditory and speech performances of CCD patients after CI usually varied (Pradhananga et al. 2015; Xia et al. 2015; Kaga et al. 2020), which probably because the distribution and number of cochlear neurons in CCD varies. So, the proper electrode placement in the cavity is very important.

However, due to the absence of modiolus in CCD, the electrode is easy into the IAC and also unstable. In addition, wrong positioning or kinking of the electrode may also occur during surgery. There have been several reports about electrode displacement in CCD's CI surgery (Ahmad and Lokman 2005; Bloom et al. 2009). To prevent this, customized electrodes, special surgical approaches, such as labyrinthotomy, and tissue filled in the cavity after electrode insertion are needed (Beltrame et al. 2013; Wei et al. 2018).

6.5 Vestibular Stimulation

For the same reason as facial nerve stimulation in CCD, the vestibular nerve could be stimulated by an electrode in the cavity. Sennaroglu et al. (2001) reported one patient with CCD occurred nystagmus when CI activated, and the MRI showed the vestibulocochlear nerve entered the cavity without dividing into cochlear and vestibular branches, therefore they thought there existed common vestibulocochlear nerve. After adjustment, there was no nystagmus 3 months later which indicated the vestibular nerve can adapt to electrical stimulation. In clinical, we should inform the audiologist of being careful of vertigo occurring during CCD patients' first cochlea programming. In our center, we also found that some CCD patients occurred slightly tilting forth and back during cochlear programming because of vestibular stimulation, and after decrease of the responsible electrodes' stimulation currents, the phenomenon disappeared.

6.6 Conclusion

CCDs have special anatomy, and CI surgery is more difficult than normal cochlea. And the common complication after CI surgery for CCD patients mainly include CSF gusher, facial nerve injury and stimulation, vestibular stimulation, and electrode displacement. But by proper preventive strategies, suitable surgical approaches and special electrodes, the complications are controllable and rarely at present.

References

Ahmad RL, Lokman S. Cochlear implantation in congenital cochlear abnormalities. Med J Malaysia. 2005;60(3):379–82.

Arimappamagan A, Sadashiva N, et al. CSF Rhinorrhea following medical treatment for Prolactinoma: management and challenges. J Neurol Surg B Skull Base. 2019;80(6):620–5.

Beltrame MA, Frau GN, et al. Double posterior labyrinthotomy technique: results in three med-El patients with common cavity. Otol Neurotol. 2005;26(2):177–82.

Beltrame MA, Birman CS, et al. Common cavity and custom-made electrodes: speech perception and audiological performance of children with common cavity implanted with a custom-made MED-EL electrode. Int J Pediatr Otorhinolaryngol. 2013;77(8):1237–43.

Bloom JD, Rizzi MD, et al. Real-time intraoperative computed tomography to assist cochlear implant placement in the malformed inner ear. Otol Neurotol. 2009;30(1):23–6.

Buchman CA, Copeland BJ, et al. Cochlear implantation in children with congenital inner ear malformations. Laryngoscope. 2004;114(2):309–16.

Cohen NL, Hoffman RA, et al. Medical or surgical complications related to the nucleus multichannel cochlear implant. Ann Otol Rhinol Laryngol Suppl. 1988;135:8–13.

Dhanasingh A, Dietz A, et al. Human inner-ear malformation types captured in 3D. J Int Adv Otol. 2019;15(1):77–82.

Farinetti A, Ben GD, et al. Cochlear implant complications in 403 patients: comparative study of adults and children and review of the literature. Eur Ann Otorhinolaryngol Head Neck Dis. 2014;131(3):177–82.

Fishman AJ, Roland JJ, et al. Fluoroscopically assisted cochlear implantation. Otol Neurotol. 2003;24(6):882–6.

Graham JM, Phelps PD, et al. Congenital malformations of the ear and cochlear implantation in children: review and temporal bone report of common cavity. J Laryngol Otol Suppl. 2000;25:1–14.

Hoffman RA, Downey LL, et al. Cochlear implantation in children with cochlear malformations. Am J Otol. 1997;18(2):184–7.

Incesulu A, Adapinar B, et al. Cochlear implantation in cases with incomplete partition type III (X-linked anomaly). Eur Arch Otorhinolaryngol. 2008;265(11):1425–30.

Kaga K, Minami S, et al. Electrically evoked ABR during cochlear implantation and postoperative development of speech and hearing abilities in infants with common cavity deformity as a type of inner ear malformation. Acta Otolaryngol. 2020;140(1):14–21.

Khan AM, Mikulec A. Cochlear implantation in the common cavity deformity. Otolaryngol Head Neck Surg. 2005;133(2):P234–4.

Kim LS, Jeong SW, et al. Cochlear implantation in children with inner ear malformations. Ann Otol Rhinol Laryngol. 2006;115(3):205–14.

Lassig AA, Zwolan TA, et al. Cochlear implant failures and revision. Otol Neurotol. 2005;26(4):624–34.

Luntz M, Balkany T, et al. Cochlear implants in children with congenital inner ear malformations. Arch Otolaryngol Head Neck Surg. 1997;123(9):974–7.

Mandour M, Elzayat S, et al. Radiological classification of the mastoid portion of the facial nerve: impact on the surgical accessibility of the round window in cochlear implantation. Acta Otolaryngol. 2021:1–4.

Manolidis S, Tonini R, et al. Endoscopically guided placement of prefabricated cochlear implant electrodes in a common cavity malformation. Int J Pediatr Otorhinolaryngol. 2006;70(4):591–6.

Masterson L, Kumar S, et al. Cochlear implant failures: lessons learned from a UK centre. J Laryngol Otol. 2012;126(1):15–21.

McElveen JJ, Carrasco VN, et al. Cochlear implantation in common cavity malformations using a transmastoid labyrinthotomy approach. Laryngoscope. 1997;107(8):1032–6.

Miyamoto RT, Robbins AJ, et al. Cochlear implantation in the Mondini inner ear malformation. Am J Otol. 1986;7(4):258–61.

Mylanus EA, Rotteveel LJ, et al. Congenital malformation of the inner ear and pediatric cochlear implantation. Otol Neurotol. 2004;25(3):308–17.

Papsin BC. Cochlear implantation in children with anomalous cochleovestibular anatomy. Laryngoscope. 2005;115(1 Pt 2 Suppl 106):1–26.

Phelps PD, King A, et al. Cochlear dysplasia and meningitis. Am J Otol. 1994;15(4):551–7.

Pradhananga RB, Thomas JK, et al. Long term outcome of cochlear implantation in five children with common cavity deformity. Int J Pediatr Otorhinolaryngol. 2015;79(5):685–9.

Romo LV, Curtin HD. Anomalous facial nerve canal with cochlear malformations. AJNR Am J Neuroradiol. 2001;22(5):838–44.

Sennaroglu L. Cochlear implantation in inner ear malformations--a review article. Cochlear Implants Int. 2010;11(1):4–41.

Sennaroglu L, Tahir E. A novel classification: anomalous routes of the facial nerve in relation to inner ear malformations. Laryngoscope. 2020;130(11):E696–703.

Sennaroglu L, Gursel B, et al. Vestibular stimulation after cochlear implantation in common cavity deformity. Otolaryngol Head Neck Surg. 2001;125(4):408–10.

Sennaroglu L, Sarac S, et al. Surgical results of cochlear implantation in malformed cochlea. Otol Neurotol. 2006;27(5):615–23.

Sennaroglu L, Atay G, et al. A new cochlear implant electrode with a "cork"-type stopper for inner ear malformations. Auris Nasus Larynx. 2014;41(4):331–6.

Tucci DL, Telian SA, et al. Cochlear implantation in patients with cochlear malformations. Arch Otolaryngol Head Neck Surg. 1995;121(8):833–8.

Wei X, Li Y, et al. Slotted labyrinthotomy approach with customized electrode for patients with common cavity deformity. Laryngoscope. 2018;128(2):468–72.

Weiss NM, Langner S, et al. Evaluating common cavity Cochlear deformities using CT images and 3D reconstruction. Laryngoscope. 2021;131(2):386–91.

Xia J, Wang W, et al. Cochlear implantation in 21 patients with common cavity malformation. Acta Otolaryngol. 2015;135(5):459–65.

Zheng Y, Schachern PA, et al. The shortened cochlea: its classification and histopathologic features. Int J Pediatr Otorhinolaryngol. 2002;63(1):29–39.

Programming Cochlear Implants for Common Cavity Deformity

7

Ying Kong, Simeng Lu, Xingmei Wei, and Yongxin Li

7.1 Programming Content

7.1.1 Measure Electrodes Impedance

Electrode impedances are mainly used to measure whether the electrode function in the cochlea is normal, and the electrode with abnormal electrode impedance (open or short) should be closed. If an electrode has abnormal behavior intermittently, it usually indicates that there will be a permanent abnormality, and special attention should be paid to the impedance of the electrode.

7.1.2 Selecting Sound Processing Strategy and Stimulus Parameters

Generally, the default parameters including sound processing strategy, stimulation mode, stimulation rate, pulse width, number of stimulation electrodes, and others

The original version of this chapter was revised. The correction to this chapter can be found at https://doi.org/10.1007/978-981-16-8217-9_11

Y. Kong (✉)
Beijing Institute of Otolaryngology, Beijing Tongren Hospital, Capital Medical University, Beijing, China

Key Laboratory of Otolaryngology Head and Neck Surgery (Capital Medical University), Ministry of Education, Beijing, China

S. Lu · X. Wei · Y. Li
Key Laboratory of Otolaryngology Head and Neck Surgery (Capital Medical University), Ministry of Education, Beijing, China

Department of Otorhinolaryngology Head and Neck Surgery, Beijing Tongren Hospital, Capital Medical University, Beijing, China are preferred when switch-on. During follow-up mapping, evaluation can be made based on the patients' feedback, impedance measurement results, and overall measurement results. The signal coding strategy and stimulation parameters can be changed when necessary(Shapiro and Bradham 2009).

7.1.3 Threshold Level Measurement

The threshold is the minimum current stimulus intensity that patients can perceive (audible). The measurement method can be selected according to the age of patients. Adults, adolescents, or older children can use the same methods as pure tone audiometry, such as raising their hands when hearing sounds. Children can use the method of pediatric behavior audiometry to obtain the threshold according to their age.

(a) Visual reinforcement audiometry (VRA): suitable for infants over 5 months old (Lidén and Kankkunen 1969).
(b) Conditioned play audiometry (CPA): suitable for children over 2 years old (Neumann et al. 2020).

For most pediatric patients, due to the lack of good auditory experience before surgery, the initial response after postoperative programming is poor, and the test results are unstable and the repeatability is poor. Therefore, audiologists with extensive experience should conduct tests for child patients. During the programming process, two audiologists need to work together, one of whom is responsible for programming the equipment and giving stimulus signals during the test. In order to reduce the interference of actions or visual cues on the test, the operator of the equipment should avoid sitting face-to-face with children but had to watch the child's movements and expressions. Another audiologist sits face-to-face with the child who is responsible for observing the child's response to the test signal and controlling the child to be in a better test state. At the same time, it is necessary to train the child to establish conditionalization to cooperate with the entire programming process. During the test, two audiologists are required to jointly judge whether the child's response is effective.

The threshold level is as accurate as possible. If the T-Level is set too low, the patient may not hear the low sound. If the T-Level is set too high, the patient may experience greater environmental noise and limited electrical stimulation dynamic range (EDR). Some devices allow the T-Level to be set to a value related to the upper-stimulation levels. At this time, it is not necessary to measure the T-level because the software can automatically set the T-level according to the upper-stimulation levels obtained by the measurement. However, if the patient reports that the auditory outcome is not good, it is still recommended to measurement the T-level.

7.1.4 Upper-Stimulation Levels

Different manufacturers have different definitions of the upper stimulus level. In the Advanced Bionics system, it is defined as the "most comfortable" current stimulation amount, which is similar to the most comfortable threshold measured in hearing aid evaluation. In Advanced Bionics cochlear implants, this parameter is usually It is called "M-level"(Lilli et al. 2020). In the MED-EL system, the upper-stimulation level is called the "maximum comfort level" (MCL) and is defined as the amount of electrical stimulation that is "loud sound and no discomfort" (Fayed et al. 2020). For the Nucleus system, the upper-stimulation level is called C-level, which is defined as the amount of electrical stimulation that the user considers "loud but comfortable"(Henkin et al. 2003).

Therefore, during the measurement, it is necessary to explain and guide patients based on the products of different manufacturers. Adults and older adolescents can be tested using the pictures of loudness scale or language expression methods. For younger infants or patients who cannot refer to pictures and expressions, behavior observation can also be used. When testing a specific electrode, the intensity of electrical stimulation can be gradually increased until the patient's loudness discomfort threshold (LDL) is reached. Once the LDL is reached, the comfort threshold can be set to the stimulation intensity below the LDL. It is reported in the literature that adult patients with CI experience have studied the LDL and comfort threshold, and found that the comfort threshold is usually above the threshold and the intensity of 70% of the dynamic range of LDL (Beattie and Warren 1982). The same results were observed by children (Holmes and Woodford 1977). This result can help audiologists initially set the upper limit of stimulation current for patients who cannot cooperate. However, due to differences between patients, the actual application must be determined through behavioral observation.

The upper-stimulation level is a very important parameter. Low setting may have a negative impact on speech recognition, voice quality, and the ability to monitor own voice. If the setting is too high, it may cause discomfort to the sound of the patient or resistance to the device, and affect speech recognition and sound quality.

For infants and young children who cannot cooperate or adults with pre-lingual deafness, the upper-stimulation level or threshold can also be estimated based on objective tests. In clinical practice, the electrically evoked stapedius reflex threshold (ESRT) is used to estimate (Battmer et al. 1990). In addition, the threshold and upper-stimulation level can be estimated by electrically evoked compound action potential (ECAP) (Polak et al. 2005). Although these objective tests can help in programming, behavioral tests are still the most basic and effective test technique to determine the best settings for CI.

7.1.5 Loudness Balancing

This test is to minimize the distortion of the original sound signal processed by programming software. A good balance of loudness between the electrodes helps patients obtain better sound quality and speech recognition ability. During the test, 2–3 adjacent electrodes are usually selected for testing. The patient needs to point out which electrode sounds louder or lighter than the others, and the audiologist should adjust it according to the patient's response. Due to the need to compare the differences in pitch and loudness between the electrodes, this test is easier for adults or older adolescents who have been using CI for a relatively long time.

7.1.6 Pitch Scaling

The implanted electrodes hover from the base of the cochlea to the top of the cochlea. The electrodes at the base of the cochlea should produce high pitch, while the electrodes near the top of the cochlea should produce low pitch. If the pitch produced by the electrodes in some parts is significantly different from the pitch that should be produced, the order of these electrodes needs to be re-adjusted.

7.1.7 Testing the MAP

After the above tests are performed, go live to allow the patient to listen to environmental sounds and speech sounds to ensure the audibility and comfort of the sound. It can be assessed by Ling's six-tone test or speech test.

7.2 Tips for Programming of Common Cavity Deformity

The content and steps of programming for patients with CCD are the same as those for other patients. But due to the structural characteristics of CCD, there are some points that are different from other patients and require attention during programming. We used MEDEL customized electrodes during the operation, which were implanted through the single-slit labyrinthotomy approach (Wei et al. 2018). Since the size of the CCD varies greatly among individuals (Dhanasingh et al. 2019), the number of electrodes located in the cavity must be clarified through postoperative images before switch-on, and the extracochlear electrodes need to be turned off. We performed the intraoperative ART test on 10 patients, and the total extraction rate was 55%, of which the extraction rate of electrodes no. 2 and 12 was 40% (8/20), and the extraction rate of electrodes no. 4 and 10 was 50% (10/20), the extraction rate of electrode no. 6 and no. 8 was 75% (15/20). The ECAP response amplitude of electrodes at different positions ranged from 50.69 to 170.3 μV, and individual differences were large. The ECAP amplitude of some children did not increase with the increase of stimulation intensity, and the response amplitude of different electrodes did not change significantly. The intraoperative ART can reflect the function of the electrode and the integrity of the entire transmission path, but it has little relevance to the parameter settings for postoperative programming. And postoperative ART is not easy to elicit for CCD patients.

For patients with CCD, the current of MCL is usually relatively high, so in the programming process, attention should be paid to whether it will cause facial nerve stimulation symptoms or non-auditory reactions. If the electrodes cause strong discomfort, they need to be turned off, or the stimulations model needs to be changed.

In some patients, it was obvious that the MCL of electrodes no. 4 to 8 were significantly lower than the other electrodes (Fig. 7.1), and a little larger MCL would cause slightly tilting forth and back or discomfort. In some patients, the MCL of no. 4 to 8 were gradually increasing with the using time and became similar to other electrodes (Fig. 7.2), but some patients' MCL of no. 4 to 8 electrodes declined with the using time (Fig. 7.3). There is no significant difference in the impedance of each electrode, and now the reason for this phenomenon has not been found. We thought it may be because electrodes no. 4 to 8 are closer to the internal auditory canal (IAC), which has more spiral ganglia at this position and more sensitive for electrical stimulation. Therefore, it is necessary to pay more attention to patient's reactions when programming electrodes no. 4 to 8, especially infants and young children, and

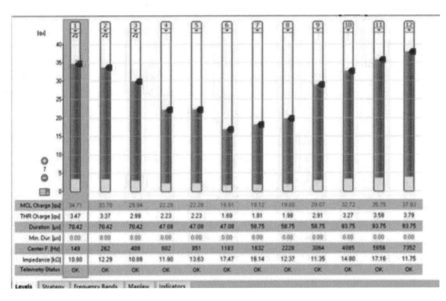

Fig. 7.1 The example of maximum comfortable level of electrodes no. 4 to 8 were significantly lower than the other electrodes

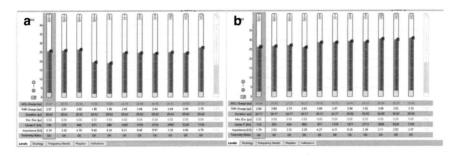

Fig. 7.2 An example of maximum comfortable level of from curved (December 2019) to flat (January 2020). (**a**) The curved maximum comfortable level in December 2019. (**b**) The flat maximum comfortable level in January 2020

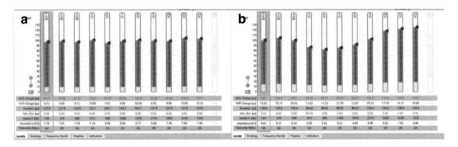

Fig. 7.3 An example of maximum comfortable level of from flat (July 2020) to curved (September 2020). (**a**) The flat maximum comfortable level in July 2020. (**b**) The curved maximum comfortable level in September 2020

careful observation of facial expressions and behavior to determine the appropriate MCL.

For further exploring the correlation among programming performance, MCL map and auditory performance, we include 25 patients (27 ears) with CCD who underwent CI using customized electrodes. The patient's uncomfortable reactions during the process of programming were recorded, such as facial nerve stimulation or slightly tilting forth and back. Due to the programming parameters coming to stable in about 6 months after switch-on, we choose the MCL at that time. Furthermore, the patients underwent auditory and speech assessments during each follow-up by means of the following scales: Categories of Auditory Performance (CAP), Speech Intelligibility Rating (SIR), Meaningful Auditor Integration Scale (for patients in the age group of 3–6 years)/Infant-Toddler Meaningful Auditor Integration Scale (for subjects <3 years of age) (MAIS/ITMAIS), and Meaningful Use of Speech Scale (MUSS). The scores obtained one, two, and three years after the surgical procedure were selected to do a comparison. The patients were divided into symptomatic and asymptomatic groups according to with or without abnormal reactions, and flat and curved groups according to the MCL.

The results showed abnormal reactions during cochlear programming in 10 ears (37%), whereas the other 17 ears (63%) did not exhibit any abnormal reaction. Among the aforementioned cases of abnormal reactions, facial nerve stimulation was observed in six cases and four displayed slightly tilting forth and back, owing to vestibular nerve stimulation. The facial nerve stimulation was mainly instigated by the no. 4 to 7 electrodes and deactivation of the responsible electrodes resulted in resolution of the symptoms. The abnormal reaction of slightly tilting forth and back was caused by the respective no. 4, no. 5, and no. 7 electrodes in three cases. The modification of electric current resulted in the resolution of symptoms in the subjects who exhibited slightly tilting forth and back. T-test showed that the average MCL in the symptomatic group was significantly smaller ($p < 0.05$), but impedance showed no significant difference (Table 7.1). There was a significant difference between the two groups in regard to the MCL of electrodes (no. 1 and nos. 3–10), which was observed to be lower in the symptomatic group compared to the asymptomatic group (Fig. 7.4). The postoperative auditory results showed that the CAP scores one year after surgery was significantly better in the symptomatic group,

Table 7.1 The sample size, average impedance, and maximum comfortable level (MCL) in the symptomatic and asymptomatic groups

Groups	asymptomatic	symptomatic	T-test value
No.(%)	17(63%)	10(37%)	–
Average impedances	7.65 ± 2.04	7.78 ± 2.17	0.03, 0.957
Average MCL	57.06 ± 11.36	36.19 ± 4.03	7.044, 0.014*

The asterisk ("*") indicates a significant difference

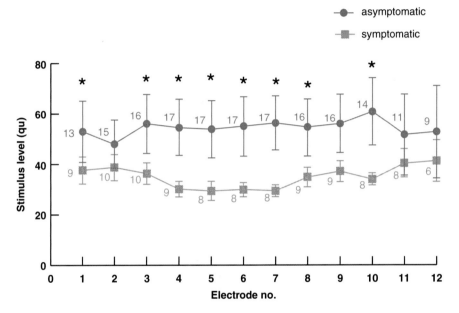

Fig. 7.4 The comparison of maximum comfortable level between asymptomatic and symptomatic groups of each electrode. The asterisk ("*") indicates a significant difference (reproduced with permission from Wei et al. 2022, Front. Neurol. 12:783225)

whereas no significant difference was observed in relation to the scores of other questionnaires (Fig. 7.5). In addition, the contour of the MCL map was flat in relation to 12 ears (44.4%) and curved in relation to 15 ears (55.6%). In the flat group, merely one ear showed an abnormal reaction during programming, whereas nine ears (69%) in the curved group were symptomatic. The average MCL was lower in the curved group than the flat group. However, the difference was not statistically significant and the magnitude of current was significantly different (Table 7.2). The present study did not observe any significant difference between the two groups with regard to the impedance of each electrode. The MCL in the flat group was higher than the curved group (Fig. 7.6). Moreover, the present study observed a significant difference between the two groups in regard to the MCL in relation to the nos. 1, 3, 4, 5, 6, and 7 electrodes ($p < 0.05$), and the flat group displayed higher. The scores of questionnaires employed to assess the outcomes one, two, and three years after surgery in the curved group were greater than the flat group. And the CAP after

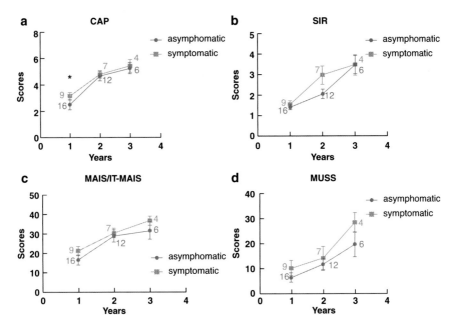

Fig. 7.5 The comparison of CAP, SIR, MAIS/IT-MAIS and MUSS between asymptomatic and symptomatic groups 1, 2, and 3 years after surgery. The asterisk ("*") indicates a significant difference. (**a**) The CAP scores. (**b**) The SIR scores. (**c**) The MAIS/IT-MAIS scors. (**d**) The MUSS scores of the asymphomatic and symptomatic groups 1,2,3 years after surgery (reproduced with permission from Wei et al. 2022, Front. Neurol. 12:783225)

Table 7.2 The sample size, average impedance, and maximum comfortable level (MCL) in the curved and flat groups

Groups	Curved	Flat	T-test value
No.(%)	15(55.6%)	12(44.4%)	–
Average impedances	7.56 ± 1.99	7.9 ± 2.19	0.306, 0.585
Average MCL	42.34 ± 5.90	58.06 ± 15.17	6.586, 0.017*

The asterisk ("*") indicates a significant difference

one year and SIR score after 3 years of curved group were significantly better than the flat group (Fig. 7.7). The results showed the differences mainly came from medial electrodes, and the outcomes of symptomatic and curved groups were better. The reason may be because of the medial electrodes adjacent to IAC, if they were adjacent to cavity wall, the MCL were lower, more spiral ganglia could be stimulated, and the outcomes were better, but the facial and vestibular nerve stimulation rate was higher.

Since the postoperative effect of CCD patients is worse than that of patients with normal cochlear structure, it is very important for the audiologist to communicate with patients and family members and establish expectations. The expected values that are taken will also have a positive impact on postoperative recovery. For

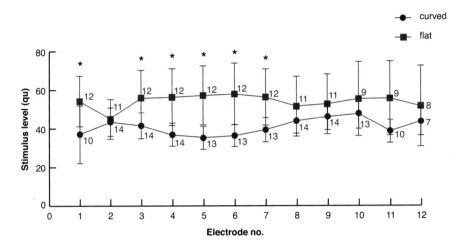

Fig. 7.6 The comparison of maximum comfortable level between curved and flat groups of each electrode. The asterisk ("*") indicates a significant difference (reproduced with permission from Wei et al. 2022, Front. Neurol. 12:783225)

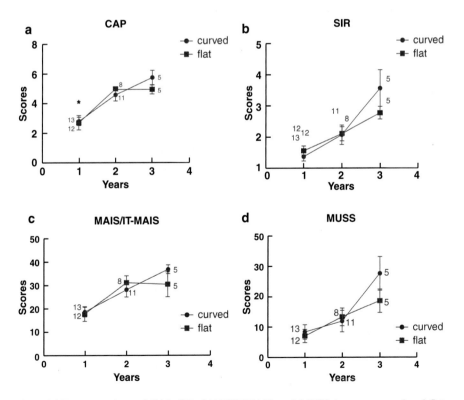

Fig. 7.7 The comparison of CAP, SIR, MAIS/IT-MAIS, and MUSS between curved and flat groups 1, 2, and 3 years after surgery. The asterisk ("*") indicates significant difference. (**a**) The CAP scores. (**b**) The SIR scores. (**c**) The MAIS/IT-MAIS scors. (**d**) The MUSS scores of the curved and flat groups 1,2,3 years after surgery (reproduced with permission from Wei et al. 2022, Front. Neurol. 12:783225)

CCD patients, the programming interval is also recommended to be shorter than other patients, such we can in time obtain the patient's MAP changes and rehabilitation efficacy.

7.3 Cases

There are 2 cases below.

7.3.1 Case 1

A male patient who was born in November 2017 had failed passing newborn hearing screening and had bilateral CCD with cochlear nerve deficiency. The right ear was implanted in July 2019, using MEDEL Mi1000 custom electrodes. During the operation, the impedance test of all electrodes was normal, and the ART test of No. 4 and No. 7 electrodes could elicit reactions.

One month after surgery, the impedance test showed that all the electrodes were normal. The postoperative CT results showed that all electrodes were implanted, and all electrodes were turned on. During the programming process, it was discovered that the body would shake slightly when the stimulation current of electrodes 4–6 was about 20 qu; therefore, the audiologist stopped increasing the stimulation current. The stimulation volume used by electrodes 4–6 was significantly lower than other electrodes (Fig. 7.8). When Go Live, the children can detect

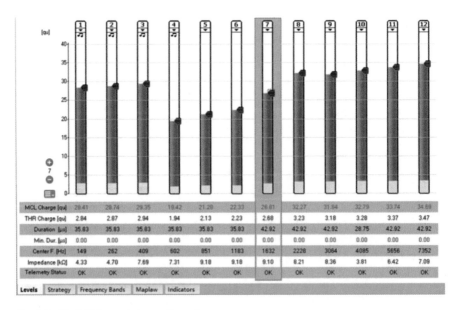

Fig. 7.8 The MAP at switch-on of case 1

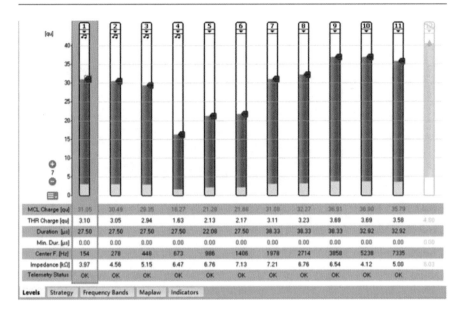

MCL Charge [qu]	31.05	30.49	29.35	16.27	21.28	21.88	31.08	32.27	26.91	36.90	35.79	
THR Charge [qu]	3.10	3.05	2.94	1.63	2.13	2.17	3.11	3.23	3.69	3.69	3.58	4.60
Duration [µs]	27.50	27.50	27.50	27.50	22.08	27.50	38.33	38.33	38.33	32.92	32.92	
Min. Dur. [µs]	0.00	0.00	0.00	0.00	0.00	0.00	0.00	0.00	0.00	0.00	0.00	0.00
Center F. [Hz]	154	278	448	673	988	1406	1978	2714	3858	5238	7335	
Impedance [kΩ]	3.97	4.56	5.15	6.47	6.76	7.13	7.21	6.76	6.54	4.12	5.00	8.03
Telemetry Status	OK	OK	OK	OK	OK	OK	OK	OK	OK	OK	OK	

Fig. 7.9 The MAP at second mapping

moderate-intensity sounds such as clapping hands and knocking on the table, and there was no uncomfortable response to loud sounds.

The second programming was one month after the switch-on, and no clear auditory response was observed on the no. 12 electrode when the stimulation level was large, so we turned off the electrode (Fig. 7.9). When Go Live, the child was able to perceive moderate-intensity ambient sounds and speech sounds, there was no uncomfortable reaction to loud sounds.

After that, the child was programmed 4 times latter, and the stimulation current and impedance of each electrode changed little and were relatively stable (Fig. 7.10). After CI was activated, he continued to perform auditory and speech rehabilitation training, and the IT-MAIS, MUSS, CAP, and SIR scales were used for assessment. Twenty months after switch-on, IT-MAIS, MUSS, CAP, and SIR reached 39, 15, 5, and 3, respectively. And the speech recognition rate of closed two-syllable words reached 63.3%. The parents are quite satisfied with the current results.

7.3.2 Case 2

A male patient who was born in April 2016 had failed to pass newborn hearing. He had bilateral CCD with bilateral vestibular and cochlear nerve deficiency, and his right side was worse development. His left ear was implanted in April 2018, using MEDEL Mi1000 custom electrodes. During the operation, all electrode impedance tests showed normal.

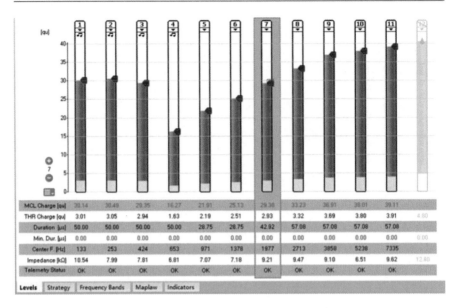

Fig. 7.10 The MAP at sixth mapping

One month after surgery, the postoperative CT showed that the no. 1 electrode was located external the cavity, and the rest electrodes were in the cavity. When the cochlear is switched on, the impedance of no. 2–12 electrodes was normal, so we turned them on. During the programming process, we found that when the stimulation current of the no. 7 electrode was about 29 qu, the children's body would slightly tilt forth and back; therefore, we stopped increasing the stimulation current. The stimulation current of no. 7 electrode was significantly lower than that of other electrodes. No clear auditory response was observed on electrode no. 11, so we turned off it. There was obvious facial nerve stimulation when the stimulation current of no. 4 electrode was around 18 qu, so we turned off it (Fig. 7.11). When Go Live, the patient was able to perceive the moderate-intensity sound of knocking on the table, he showed no uncomfortable response to loud sounds.

In the second mapping, no auditory response was observed on the no. 2 electrode even the stimulation current was large, so we turned it off (Fig. 7.12). When Go Live, he was able to perceive moderate-intensity ambient sounds and speech sounds, there was no uncomfortable reaction to loud sounds. Afterward, his left ear was programming as scheduled, and we found that no. 12 electrode was no clear auditory response to large stimulus current, and it was turned off (Fig. 7.13). The child continued to undergo auditory and speech rehabilitation training. After 6 months of switching-on, IT-MAIS, MUSS, CAP, and SIR reached 26, 19, 4, and 2, respectively.

His right ear was implanted in November 2018, using MEDEL Mi1000 custom electrodes. During surgery, all electrode impedance tests showed normal.

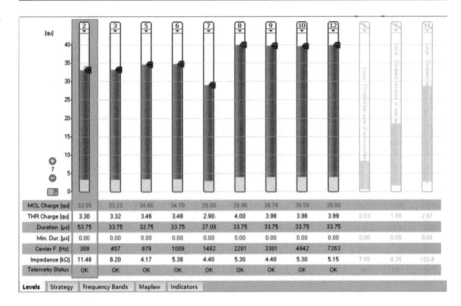

Fig. 7.11   The MAP of first mapping after the left ear implanted

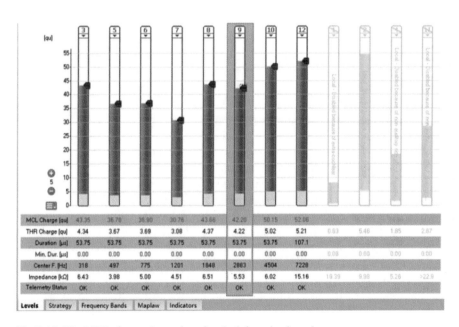

Fig. 7.12   The MAP of second mapping after the left ear implanted

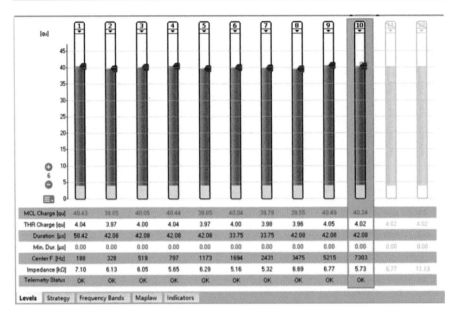

	1	2	3	4	5	6	7	8	9	10		
MCL Charge [qu]	40.43	39.85	40.05	40.44	39.85	40.04	39.79	39.55	40.49	40.24		
THR Charge [qu]	4.04	3.97	4.00	4.04	3.97	4.00	3.98	3.96	4.05	4.02	4.02	4.02
Duration [µs]	50.42	42.08	42.08	42.08	42.08	33.75	33.75	42.08	42.08	42.08		
Min. Dur. [µs]	0.00	0.00	0.00	0.00	0.00	0.00	0.00	0.00	0.00	0.00	0.00	0.00
Center F. [Hz]	188	328	519	797	1173	1694	2431	3475	5215	7303		
Impedance [kΩ]	7.10	6.13	6.05	5.65	6.29	5.16	5.32	6.69	6.77	5.73	6.77	11.13
Telemetry Status	OK	OK	OK	OK	OK	OK	OK	OK	OK	OK		

Fig. 7.13 The MAP of seventh mapping after the left ear implanted

One month after surgery, the right side was switched-on. After surgery, temporal bone CT showed that all the electrodes were implanted in the cavity. The impedances of all electrodes were normal when CI was activated. During the programming, it was found that no. 11 and 12 electrodes showed no clear auditory response to high stimulation current, so they were turned off (Fig. 7.14). When Go Live, he can perceive the sound of drums, clapping, and knocking on the table, and he showed no uncomfortable reaction to loud sounds.

During the second and third mapping after the second surgery, electrodes 6 to 10 all showed different degrees of facial nerve stimulation symptoms, so we reduced stimulation current (Fig. 7.15). During the sixth programming, electrodes no. 1 and 4 did not respond clearly to loud sounds and they were turned off (Fig. 7.16).

The patient received hearing and speech rehabilitation training after CI on the right side. Thirty months after the switch-on, IT-MAIS, MUSS, CAP, and SIR reached 38, 31, 6, and 4, respectively. After 36 months of the switch-on, the closed two-syllable speech recognition rate in a quiet environment was 95%, and the short sentence recognition rate was 100%.

Before surgery, the child cannot walk alone and was easy to fall down. After his left ear was implanted, he could walk himself, but was unstable. After the right CI, after sensory integration training, he could walk independently and stably one year after the second surgery, and he could run and jump two years after surgery. The child can now engage in daily dialogue and communication and has a strong sense of active communication. The parents are very satisfied with the postoperative outcomes.

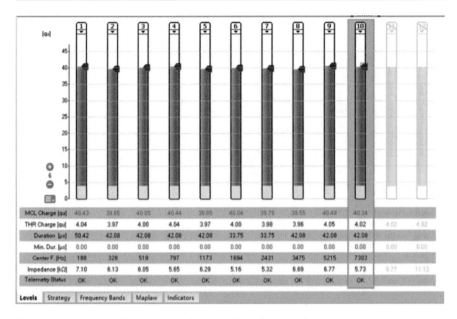

Fig. 7.14   The MAP of first mapping after the right ear implanted

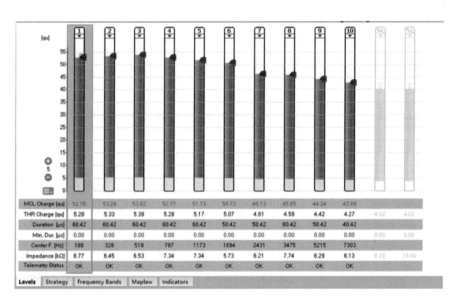

Fig. 7.15   The MAP of second mapping after the right ear implanted

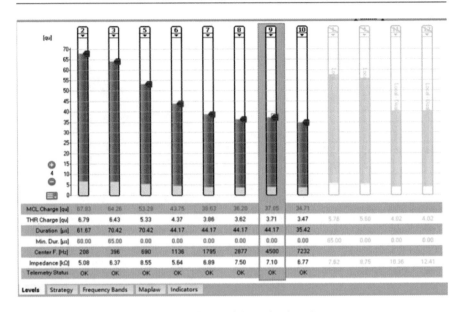

Fig. 7.16 The MAP of sixth mapping after the right ear implanted

References

Battmer RD, Laszig R, et al. Electrically elicited stapedius reflex in cochlear implant patients. Ear Hear. 1990;11(5):370–4.

Beattie RC, Warren VG. Relationships among speech threshold, loudness discomfort, comfortable loudness, and PB max in the elderly hearing impaired. Am J Otol. 1982;3(4):353.

Dhanasingh A, et al. Human inner-ear malformation types captured in 3D. J Int Adv Otol. 2019;15(1):77–82.

Fayed EA, Zaghloul HS, et al. Electrode impedance changes over time in MED El cochlear implant children recipients: relation to stimulation levels and behavioral measures. Cochlear Implants Int. 2020;21(4):1–6.

Henkin Y, Kaplan-Neeman R, et al. Changes over time in electrical stimulation levels and electrode impedance values in children using the nucleus 24M cochlear implant. Int J Pediatr Otorhinolaryngol. 2003;67(8):873–80.

Holmes DW, Woodford CM. Acoustic reflex threshold and loudness discomfort level: relationships in children with profound hearing losses. J Am Audiol Soc. 1977;2(6):193–6.

Lidén G, Kankkunen A. Visual reinforcement audiometry. Acta Otolaryngol. 1969;67(2–6):281–92.

Lilli G, Lenarz T, et al. Cochlear Implantation with the new Advanced Bionics SlimJ electrode in children. Abstract- und Posterband—91. Jahresversammlung der Deutschen Gesellschaft für HNO-Heilkunde, Kopf- und Hals-Chirurgie e.V., Bonn—Welche Qualität macht den Unterschied; 2020.

Neumann S, Smith J, et al. Conditioned play audiometry: keeping the play in CPA! Hear J. 2020;73:14–6.

Polak M, Hodges A, et al. ECAP, ESR and subjective levels for two different nucleus 24 electrode arrays. Otol Neurotol. 2005;26(4):639–45.

Shapiro WH, Bradham TS. Cochlear implant programming. Otolaryngol Clin N Am. 2009;45(1):111–27.

Wei X, Li Y, et al. Slotted labyrinthotomy approach with customized electrode for patients with common cavity deformity. Laryngoscope. 2018;128(2) https://doi.org/10.1002/lary.26627.

Outcomes of Common Cavity Deformity After Cochlear Implantation

8

Xingmei Wei, Shujin Xue, Yongxin Li, Lifang Zhang, Biao Chen, Mengge Yang, and Simeng Lu

8.1 Speech Perception Assessment

8.1.1 Parent Report Scales

For patients who cannot cooperation with behavioral measures of speech perception, questionnaires can be useful in assessing their auditory development. There are some commonly used questionnaires listed as follows:

The meaningful auditory integration scale (MAIS) (Robbins et al. 1991) (for ages 3–6 years) and infants and toddlers meaningful auditory integration scale (IT-MAIS) (for ages<3 year) (Mcconkey Robbins et al. 2004) are two of the most commonly used questionnaires. They were initially developed for parents and educators to evaluate the child's responses to their daily environment sounds. The MAIS and IT-MAIS both include 10 questions, and each question receives a score of 0–4 depending on how frequently the child demonstrates the behavior. MAIS mainly assess the use of cochlear device (questions 1–2), detection ability for sound (questions 3–6) and understanding ability for sound (question 7–10). And for IT-MAIS, only the first two questions are different, which evaluate the children's vocal behavior.

The Meaningful Use of Speech Scale (MUSS) (Crosson 1992) is another scale to assess children's speech ability with CI, and it consists of 11 questions, and each question also contains five levels of 0–4 scores. The MUSS mainly

X. Wei (✉) · S. Xue · Y. Li · L. Zhang · B. Chen · M. Yang · S. Lu
Department of Otorhinolaryngology Head and Neck Surgery, Beijing Tongren Hospital, Capital Medical University, Beijing, China

Key Laboratory of Otolaryngology Head and Neck Surgery (Capital Medical University), Ministry of Education, Beijing, China assesses vocal control (questions 1–3), use of speech without gesture or sign (questions 4–7) and use of communication strategies in everyday situations (questions 8–11).

The Categories of Auditory Performance (CAP) score (Archbold et al. 1995) is used worldwide to evaluate the subjects' auditory performance in their daily life, including the perception of natural environment and speech sounds. The CAP ranges from 0 to 7 scores, which increase with the development of auditory level. The Speech Intelligibility Rating (SIR) scale (Allen et al. 2001) is for evaluation of subjects' speech performance and includes 1–5 grades from low to high. The SIR can quickly help us assess subjects' language comprehension based on their daily routine. The CAP and SIR can obtain from their parents or rehabilitation workers who are familiar with the auditory impaired subjects.

8.1.2 Detection Discrimination Recognition Comprehension

The auditory and speech discrimination and recognition ability of infants and little children are not easy to assess. In clinical, we usually by techniques, such as behavioral observation audiometry and visual reinforcement audiometry (VRA)to assess their sound detection abilities. VRA was mainly used in prelinguistic infants with normal hearing to assess their ability to discriminate speech features or speech sounds (Kuhl 1979). There was no report about VRA used for CCD patients, and we will not describe it in detail.

8.1.3 Speech Perception Tests

According to stimulation presentation voice, the speech perception tests can classify into live voice and recorded. The live-voice tests are mainly used for very young children, but it is not convenient for longitudinal comparisons within a given child or cross-sectional comparisons across children, and the use of live-voice tests was limited. The recorded tests can be used for children above 3 or 4 years old. For example, Kindergarten Word List (PBK) (Haskins 1949) and the Hearing in Noise Test for Children (HINT-C) (Soli et al. 2002) are recorded test.

According to stimulation presentation mode, the speech perception tests include auditory-only format or an auditory-plus-visual format, and the former one is commonly used. In some difficult listening situations, the visual cues can help increase response ability (Sumby and W 1954).

More usually, the speech perception tests are used according to response format, which include closed-set tests and open-set tests. They should be chosen according to children's age, attention span and speech intelligibility skills. In closed-set tests, patients were asked to point to one of the given series of pictures or objects, which helps maintain interest and attention in the task and need not vocabulary demands. Most closed-set tests assess perception of isolated words, although tests of closed-set sentence recognition are available. Closed-set tests are mainly for young children or those who cannot provide intelligible verbal responses, as in the early stages of CI use. The common used closed-set speech perception tests are word intelligibility by picture identification (WIPI) (Ross and Lerman 1970), pediatric speech intelligibility (PSI) (Jerger et al. 1980), Children's Realistic Intelligibility and Speech Perception (CRISP) (Litovsky and Ruth 2005),CRISP-Jr (Garadat and Litovsky 2007), early speech perception (ESP) (Genovese et al. 1995), mandarin early speech perception test (MESP) (Zheng et al. 2009), and so on. Open-set tests require the subjects to produce some sort of verbal, written, or signed response. Open-set tests include word and sentence recognition tests. The common used open-set tests are multisyllabic lexical neighborhoods test (MLNT), Mandarin lexical neighborhood (MLNT), lexical neighborhoods (LNT), phonetically based kindergarten (PBK) (Haskins 1949), Bamford-Kowal-Bench (BKB) (Bench et al. 1979), hearing in noise test for children (HINT-C) (Soli et al. 2002), AV-LNST (Holt et al. 2011), Pediatric AzBio (Spahr et al. 2012), MLST-C (Kirk et al. 2012), Test of Auditory Comprehension (TAC) (Davis 1977), Glendonald Auditory Screening Procedure (GASP) test (Chathurika 2016), Mandarin lexical neighborhood test (MLNT) (Zhang et al. 2009), Mandarin speech perception (MSP) (Ying et al. 2015), and so on.

8.2   Auditory and Speech Outcomes of CCD

Researches on the auditory and speech outcomes of cochlear implants in children with CCD showed that although outcomes of CCD are generally worse than those with normal inner ear structures or mild deformities, it is certain that most CCD patients can regain hearing through cochlear implant (Pakdaman et al. 2011; Pradhananga et al. 2015). For the auditory and speech assessment of CCD patients, there are many questionnaire results reported in the literatures, and some studies include the results of some open or closed-set tests.

8.2.1   Overall Auditory and Speech Outcomes

As early as 2004, Ahmad et al. performed CI surgery on a 2-years-old CCD patient through a cochleostomy approach, and the child responded to environmental sounds 1 year after the surgery, but there was no speech improvement (Ahmad and Lokman 2005). In 2005, Papsin et al. conducted a study on the postoperative results of CI in 103 patients with cochlear malformations, two closed-set tests were used, which included the TAC and WIPI, and three open-set tests, the GASP, PBK-word, and PBK-phoneme were also used. The results showed that eight patients with CCD performed more poorly than other groups, such as incomplete partition and vestibular aqueduct enlargement (Papsin 2005), and only two of eight CCD patients can complete closed or open-set speech perception tests. Buchman (2004) also observed this phenomenon. They analyzed 28 patients with inner ear deformities and compared them with the closed-set test ESP and the open-set test PBK, found that the more severe the deformity, the worse the effect. Among them, one patient with CCD can only develop some closed-set recognition. But there are different conclusions. For example, in 2010, Dettman and Sadeghi-Barzalighi et al. followed up 48 patients with different types of inner ear malformations, 5 of which were CCD (Dettman et al. 2010). They used the open-set speech test BKB, 3 of the CCD patients achieved open speech recognition, with an average recognition rate of 56.3%, and the results showed no significant difference with patients of other deformities in speech outcomes, but they found that the length of electrode implantation significant influenced the results. Therefore, they believe that the number of activated electrodes had a more significant impact on speech outcomes. The different conclusions among those researches may be related to the variety of the sample size of various deformities in different studies, and the sample size of each deformity is limited.

8.2.2 Longitudinal CCD's Auditory and Speech Outcomes

Recently, the long-term outcomes of CCD patients after CI were valued. In 2011, Ahn et al. completed a long-term follow-up of 11 CCD patients with CI and found that their auditory and speech outcomes were still improving 3 years after surgery (Ahn et al. 2011). The research's average follow-up time was 80.5 ± 24.1 months and they used IT-MAIS, CAP, SIR and open-set one and two-syllable word recognition tests to evaluate the outcomes. SIR increased from 0 before surgery to 3 at 48 months after surgery, MAIS increased from 0.4 to 87.9%, and CAP increased from 0.9 to 4.7. After 48 months, the score open-set speech test did not improve a lot. At 48 months after surgery, the monosyllable improved from 0 to 24.1%, and the dissyllable improved from 0 to 38.7%. There are long-term follow-up studies with a large sample size have shown that children who underwent CI surgery at an early age (<3 years) have a rapid improvement in CAP score within 24 months after surgery, reaching 6 at 24 months, and the SIR score improved quickly between 12 and 24 months, reaching 3–4 at 24 months after surgery (Guo et al. 2020). This demonstrates that the postoperative speech improvement of CCD patients takes more time than that of CI patients with normal cochlear structure.

8.2.2.1 Comparison with Normal Cochlea

For further comparison, in 2015, Xia et al. (2015) carried out a long-term follow-up of 21 CCD patients and matched same number of patients without inner ear malformations as the control group. Regular follow-ups were used as MESP, open-set auditory speech perception with MLNT-Monosyllable and MLNT-Disyllable, CAP and SIR at 1, 2, 3, 4, 12, 18, 24, 36 months. The results showed that only 50% of the CCD patients could finish the open-set speech perception. The questionnaires or speech perception tests all showed CCD group were developed slower than the control group, and the scores were all lower for CCD group. In the same year, Pradhananga et al. (2015) reported the follow-up results of the auditory and speech outcomes of 5 CCD patients 3 years after surgery. They were followed up regularly with CAP, SIR, MAIS, and MUSS questionnaires, and the results showed that the

CAP score increased from an average of 0.4 to 3.4 after 1 year, and then reached 5.0 after 3 years. SIR increased from 1 to 2.4 after 1 year, and to 3.2 after 3 years. The average score of MAIS after 3 years is 32.4, and the average score of MUSS is 26.4. The results showed the scores of CAP and MAIS improved more significantly than SIR and MUSS, and the improvement of SIR is slower than CAP. We can conclude that the improvement of speech ability is more difficult and slower than the auditory ability. Later, more studies conducted a long-term follow-up and analyzed the relationship between auditory and speech outcomes. Beltrame et al. followed up 19 CCD patients who underwent CI for a long time. They used CAP, SIR, and Ling 6-Sound test to evaluate the postoperative outcomes and found that the auditory and speech ability still improved until 5 years after surgery (Fig. 8.1). The relationship analysis between CAP and SIR scores showed that they are significantly related at 4 years after surgery (Beltrame et al. 2013), which demonstrated that auditory and speech ability need a long time to achieve consistent development after CI.

8.2.2.2 Comparison with Other Malformation

Someone also compared the results of long-term follow-up results after CI among different inner ear malformations. A meta-analysis of 213 patients with inner ear malformations from 59 studies was done by Farhood and concluded that long-term

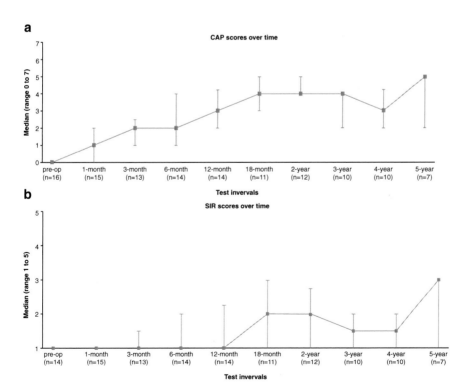

Fig. 8.1 The pictures are reproduced with permission from Beltrame et al. 2013. (**a**) Median CAP scores over the tested period. (**b**) Median SIR scores over the tested period

postoperative outcomes of CCD and cochlear hypoplasia (CH) are worse than incomplete partition type 2 (IP-II) patients, which were tested by both closed or open speech tests (Farhood et al. 2017). The results concluded that the severity of inner ear deformity affect the postoperative outcomes, and CCD is worse than IP-II but better than CH.

8.3 Longitudinal CCD's Auditory and Speech Outcomes of Our Research

In order to further study the long-term postoperative auditory and speech outcomes of CCD patients, this chapter introduces the outcomes of our center's long-term follow-up of CCD with a relative larger sample size. We conducted a long-term follow-up by questionnaire for 26 children with CCD and 59 children in the control group. The methods and results are introduced as follow.

Perform CAP, SIR, MUSS, MAIS (IT-MAIS) questionnaire assessments for children at 1, 3, 6, 9 months, 1, 1.5, 2, 3 years after cochlear switch-on. For MAIS/IT-MAIS and MUSS assessment questionnaires, we convert the actual score of the questionnaire into a percentage as the final statistical data, that is, MAIS/IT-MAIS score percentage (%) = MAIS/IT-MAIS actual score/40 points * 100%, MUSS score percentage (%) = MUSS actual score/40 * 100%.

The general conditions of these patients are shown in Table 8.1.

8.3.1 Hearing Results

Both the MAIS/IT-MAIS and the CAP assess the auditory ability. The results showed that for CCD patients, the percentage of MAIS/IT-MAIS scores and CAP scores both increase with the follow-up time. There were significant differences in each stage of growth ($P < 0.05$). This demonstrates that for patients with CCD, the auditory outcome after CI has increased significantly with the follow-up time within 18 months after switch-on. However, compared with the control group, the CCD scores were lower than those of the control group (Fig. 8.2). Because some of the data were not normal distribution, we performed non-parametric tests on the four scale scores of the two groups. The median and statistical analysis results of each group are shown in Table 8.2. Figure 8.2 shows that the average scores of MAIS/IT-MAIS (Fig. 8.2) and CAP (Fig. 8.2b) in the control group increased with the

Table 8.1 General conditions

Group	Gender Male	Female	Average implantation age (x ± SD)	Average follow-up time (months)	Maximum follow-up time (months)
CCD	11	12	27.65 ± 17.30	17	48
Control group	31	28	29.00 ± 20.41	28	48

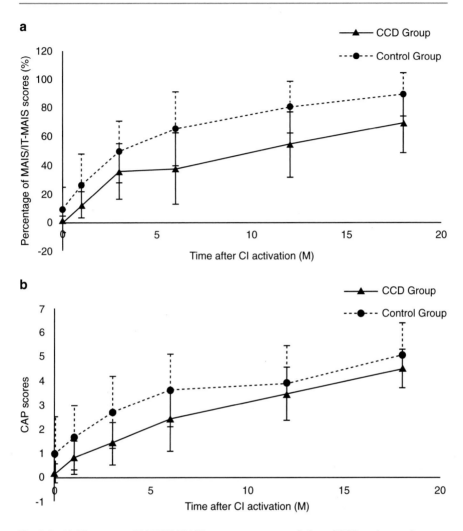

Fig. 8.2 (**a**) The average MAIS/IT-MAIS score percentage variation of CCD and control groups over time. (**b**) The average CAP score percentage variation of CCD and control groups over time

follow-up time, but the increase was faster within the first 6 months and became slower after 6 months. Although the CCD group is also gradually increasing, the average score percentage of MAIS/IT-MAIS has increased faster within the first 3 months than the second 3 months, and the average score of CAP scale increased faster within the first 6 months than the second 6 months. Compared with the control group, the percentage of MAIS/IT-MAIS scores in the CCD group was lower at all follow-up time except for 0 months after switch-on, and the difference was significant. The median CAP score of the CCD group was lower than that of the control group at 3, 6, and 12 months after switch-on. The difference between the two groups was significant at 1, 3, and 6 months. In this study, 66.67% of the children with

Table 8.2 (a) Comparison of median percentage of MAIS/ITMAIS scores between the CCD group and the control group after surgery (%, M[P25, P75]) (b) Comparison of median postoperative CAP scores between the CCD group and the control group (scores, M[P25, P75])

	0 M	1 M	3 M	6 M	12 M	18 M
(a)						
CCD group	0[0,0]	10[5,16.25]	31.25[19.375,46.875]	38.75[13.75,53.75]	50[37.5,77.5]	77.5[47.5,90]
Control group	0[0,12.5]	17.5[10,41.25]	48.75[30,61.875]	72.5[53.75,85]	87.5[70,95]	100[81.25,100]
P value	0.143	0.028	0.039	0.002	0.000	0.004
(b)						
CCD group	0[0,0]	1[0,1]	2[1,2]	2[2,3]	3[3,4]	5[4,5]
Control group	0[0,1.25]	1[1,2]	3[2,4]	4[3,5]	4[3,5]	5[4.5,6]
P value	0.064	0.013	0.001	0.012	0.195	0.123

CCD reached a CAP score of 5 by 18 months, which means they can understand commonly used phrases without the help of lip reading, but 16.67% of children can only achieve a score of 3 which means they only can identify environmental sounds. At 18 months after switch-on, the scores of children with CCD on the MAIS/IT-MAIS questionnaire ranged from 16 to 37 points. For four children who were followed up for 3 years, only one reached full score of IT -MAIS at 3 years after surgery.

8.3.2   Speech Results

MUSS can be used to assess the speech ability of children after CI, and SIR is used to assess the speech intelligibility of children. The research results of our center showed that the speech outcomes of children with CCD have gradually increased after surgery. The increase trend is shown in Fig. 8.3. The speech ability growth trend is relatively slow within 6 months after switch-on, and there is a significant growth trend between 6 and 12 months, which were consistent with the control group, but the scores are lower than those of the control group. The score comparison of scores between the two groups is shown in Table 8.3. The results showed that there is no statistical difference in MUSS between the two groups, while SIR scores are significantly different between groups at 1, 3, 6, 12, and 18 months. The difference in SIR is more obvious than that of MUSS, which may be because the MUSS questionnaire is used to evaluate the children's speech ability through three aspects: pronunciation behavior, oral communication and interpretation skills (Umat et al. 2010), the subjects in this study were all young and did not show significant

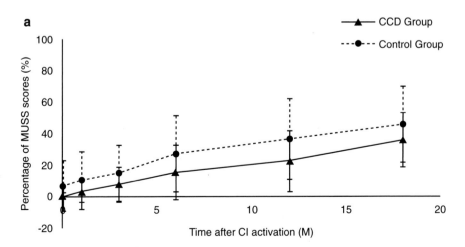

Fig. 8.3 (**a**) The average MUSS score percentage variation of CCD and control groups over time. (**b**) The average SIR score percentage variation of CCD and control groups over time

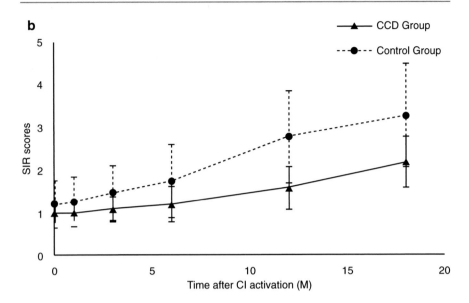

Fig. 8.3 (continued)

differences in oral communication and interpretation skills. The SIR reflects the overall level of the children's speech ability, so the differences are more significant.

8.3.3 Comparison of Hearing and Speech Perception

For the comparison between auditory and speech abilities, in this study, the median and interquartile percentages of MAIS/IT-MAIS scores for children in the CCD group were 77.5[47.5,90], CAP is 5[4,5], the MUSS score percentage is 36.25[27.5,44.375], and the SIR is 2[2,2.5]. The results showed that the scores improvement of auditory ability are more significantly than speech ability, which indicate the auditory development of CCD patients after CI is better than the speech development.

8.3.4 Correlation of Hearing and Speech Perception

To demonstrate the correlation between auditory and speech outcomes, Spearman's test was used to analyze the correlation between CAP and SIR as well as MAIS/IT-MAIS and MUSS at 1, 3, 6, 12, and 18 months after switch-on. It showed that there was no significant correlation between CAP and SIR, while MAIS/IT-MAIS and MUSS have a significant correlation at 1, 6, and 18 months. The correlation analysis scatter diagram is shown in Fig. 8.4. The possible reason for no

Table 8.3 (a) Comparison of the median postoperative MUSS score percentage between the CCD group and the control group (%, M[P25, P75]) (b) Comparison of median postoperative SIR scores between the CCD group and the control group (points, M [P25, P75])

	0 M	1 M	3 M	6 M	12 M	18 M
(a)						
CCD	0[0,0]	0[0,3.125]	3.75[0,12.5]	8.75[1.875,25.625]	15[10,35]	36.25[27.5,44.375]
Control	0[0,2.5]	0[0,15]	10[0,22.5]	17.5[9.375,45.625]	37.5[15,60]	47.5[26.25,65]
P value	0.128	0.159	0.124	0.074	0.061	0.294
(b)						
CCD	1[1,1]	1[1,1]	1[1,1]	1[1,1]	2[1,2]	2[2,2.5]
Control	1[1,1]	1[1,1]	1[1,2]	2[1,2]	3[2,3]	3[3,4]
P value	0.057	0.023	0.009	0.009	0.000	0.004

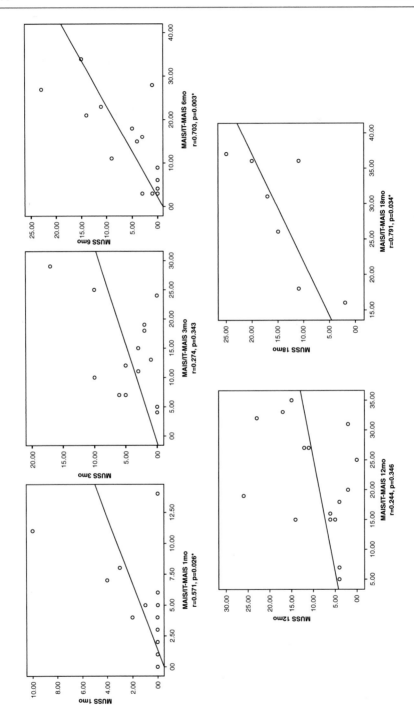

Fig. 8.4 Correlation analysis between MAIS/IT-MAIS and MUSS at 1, 3, 16, 12, and 18 months after switch-on in CCD patients. There are significant correlations at 1, 6, and 18 months ($p < 0.05$)

significant correlation between CAP and SIR is that the follow-up time is not long enough, and the SIR score needs a relative long time to develop. According to the previous study, the SIR score of CCD patients showed an increase until 1 year after surgery, and the correlation between CAP and SIR scores did not show until 4 years after surgery (Beltrame et al. 2013). The correlation between MUSS and MAIS is significant may be due to they are more detailed than SIR and CAP and can reflect smaller progress. The correlation at 1 month may be because they both are poor, and 6 months is the intersection time of the growth trend of MUSS and MAIS. MAIS grows rapidly in the first 3 months and slowly in the next 3 months, while MUSS begins to increase significantly at 6 months. Therefore, the trend of MUSS at 6 months catches up with MAIS and there is a correlation. At 18 months, both achieved better results, so there is a significant correlation. With the increase of sample size and the refinement of evaluation tools, the relationship between postoperative auditory and speech outcomes of CCD patients will be further revealed. This study needs to further increase the follow-up time, sample size and speech assessment tools to better summarize the postoperative outcomes of CCD patients.

8.3.5 Speech Perception Tests

With hearing and speech abilities' development, when the CCD patients can cooperate with closed-set or open-set speech perception tests, we evaluate their ability. Standards and Methods of Auditory & Language Skill Assessment closed-set word lists and the Disyllabic Lexical Neighborhood Test in Mandarin Chinese (Mandarin LNT and MLNT) are used.

The results of five children who underwent CI and can participate in speech perception tests are listed below. All children had bilateral CCD. Children's demographic history and results from the most recent test interval are shown in Table 8.4. All children were unable to obtain closed-set speech perception ability before CI. The range of CI use duration was from 1 to 5 years. Their best closed-set word test scores ranged from 33.5 to 100%. For the child who achieved a score was above 70%, MLNT word test underwent and achieved 65%. The results showed that CCD patients can achieve speech discrimination, and the one with bilateral CI can finish

Table 8.4 Demographics and speech perception tests of children with CCD

Case	Gender	Implanted Ear	Age of CI	Duration of use	Closed-set word test score	open-set word test score
1	M	L	1y1m	3y2m	33.30%	/
2	M	R	9m	3y4m	43.30%	/
3	F	L	1y	1y	60%	/
4	M	R	1y9 m	1y9 m	63.30%	/
5	M	R	2y8m	4y11m	100%	65%
		L	3y	4y7m		

CI cochlear implantation, *y* year, *m* month

open-set speech test, which imply us that even for CCD, bilateral implantation can make a big benefit. The long-term and big sample speech perception results will be followed.

8.4 Conclusion

The postoperative speech outcome assessments methods include questionnaires and closed-set and open-set speech tests. For CCD, the postoperative outcomes of CI were worse than that of patients without inner ear deformity or with mild deformity. Only a small number of patients could obtain open speech ability, and the improvement of postoperative auditory speech result was slower than that of patients without deformity and needed a longer time to achieve a better outcome. The development of auditory result was better than speech result, while the two showed a positive correlation with the increase of follow-up time.

References

Ahmad RL, Lokman S. Cochlear implantation in congenital cochlear abnormalities. Med J Malays. 2005;60(3):379.

Ahn JH, Lim HW, et al. Hearing improvement after cochlear implantation in common cavity malformed cochleae: long-term follow-up results. Acta Otolaryngol. 2011;131(9):908–13.

Allen C, Nikolopoulos TP, et al. Reliability of a rating scale for measuring speech intelligibility after Pediatric Cochlear implantation. Otol Neurotol. 2001;22(5):631.

Archbold S, Lutman ME, et al. Categories of auditory performance. Ann Otol Rhinol Laryngol Suppl. 1995;166:312–4.

Beltrame MA, Birman CS, et al. Common cavity and custom-made electrodes: speech perception and audiological performance of children with common cavity implanted with a custom-made MED-EL electrode. Int J Pediatr Otorhinolaryngol. 2013;77(8):1237–43.

Bench J, Kowal S, et al. The Bkb (Bamford-Kowal-Bench) sentence lists for partially-hearing children. Br J Audiol. 1979;13(3):108–12.

Buchman C. Cochlear implantation in children with congenital inner ear malformations. Laryngoscope. 2004:114.

Chathurika LKE. Developing the Kelaniya Monosyllabic—Trochee—Polysyllabic test (MTP) and Glendonald Auditory Screening Procedure (GASP) for Sinhala-speaking children. 2016.

Crosson J. Meaningful use of speech scale: application to orally educated hearing-impaired children. 1992.

Davis JM. Reliability of hearing-impaired Children's responses to Oral and Total presentations of the test of auditory comprehension of language. J Speech Hear Disord. 1977;42(4):520–7.

Dettman S, Sadeghi-Barzalighi A, et al. Cochlear implants in forty-eight children with cochlear and/or vestibular abnormality. Audiol Neurotol. 2010;16(4):222–32.

Farhood Z, Nguyen SA, et al. Cochlear implantation in inner ear malformations: systematic review of speech perception outcomes and intraoperative findings. Otolaryngol Head Neck Surg. 2017;156(3) https://doi.org/10.1177/0194599817696502.

Garadat SN, Litovsky RY. Speech intelligibility in free field: spatial unmasking in preschool children. J Acoust Soc Am. 2007;121(2):1047–55.

Genovese E, Orzan E, et al. Speech perception test in Italian language for profoundly deaf children. Acta Otorhinolaryngol Ital. 1995;15(5):383–90.

Guo Q, Lyu J, et al. The development of auditory performance and speech perception in CI children after long-period follow up. Am J Otolaryngol. 2020;41(4):102466.

Haskins HL. A phonetically balanced test of speech discrimination for children. Master's Thesis; 1949.

Holt RF, Kirk KI, et al. Assessing multimodal spoken word-in-sentence recognition in children with normal hearing and children with cochlear implants. J Speech Lang Hearing Res. 2011;54(2):632–57.

Jerger S, Lewis S, et al. Pediatric speech intelligibility test. I. Generation of test materials. Int J Pediatr Otorhinolaryngol. 1980;2(3):217–30.

Kirk KI, Prusick L, et al. Assessing spoken word recognition in children who are deaf or hard of hearing: a translational approach. J Am Acad Audiol. 2012;23(6):464–75.

Kuhl PK. Speech perception in early infancy: perceptual constancy for spectrally dissimilar vowel categories. J Acoust Soc Am. 1979;66(S1):1668–79.

Litovsky, Ruth Y. Speech intelligibility and spatial release from masking in young children. J Acoust Soc Am. 2005;117(5):3091–9.

Mcconkey Robbins A, Koch DB, et al. Effect of age at Cochlear implantation on auditory skill development in infants and toddlers. Arch Otolaryngol Head Neck Surg. 2004;130(5):570–4.

Pakdaman MN, Herrmann BS, et al. Cochlear implantation in children with anomalous Cochleovestibular anatomy. Otolaryngol Head Neck Surg. 2011;

Papsin B. Cochlear implantation in children with anomalous chochleovestibular anatomy. Laryngoscope. 2005:115.

Pradhananga RB, Thomas JK, et al. Long term outcome of cochlear implantation in five children with common cavity deformity. Int J Pediatr Otorhinolaryngol. 2015;79(5):685–9.

Robbins AM, Renshaw JJ, et al. Evaluating meaningful auditory integration in profoundly hearing-impaired children. Am J Otol. 1991;12(Suppl (3)):144.

Ross M, Lerman J. A picture identification test for hearing-impaired children. J Speech Hear Res. 1970;13(1):44–53.

Soli SD, Vermiglio A, et al. Development of the hearing in noise test (HINT) in Spanish. Acoustical Society of America Journal. 2002;112(5):2384.

Spahr AJ, Dorman MF, et al. Development and validation of the AzBio sentence lists. Ear & Hearing. 2012;33(1):112–7.

Sumby, W H. Visual contribution to speech intelligibility in noise. J Acoust Soc Am. 1954;26(2):212–5.

Umat C, Hufaidah KS, et al. Auditory Functionality and Early Use of Speech in a Group of Pediatric Cochlear Implant Users. Medical Journal of Malaysia. 2010;65(1):7–13.

Xia J, Wang W, et al. Cochlear implantation in 21 patients with common cavity malformation. Acta Otolaryngol. 2015;135(5):459–65.

Ying S, Li Y, et al. The preliminary analysis of the list equivalency of disyllabic materials for mandarin speech perception test in Cochlear implant users. J Audiol Speech Pathol. 2015;

Zhang N, Sheng YQ, et al. The development of mandarin monosyllable lexical Neighborhood test. J Audiol Speech Pathol. 2009;35(10):31–6.

Zheng Y, Meng ZL, et al. Development of the mandarin early speech perception test: children with normal hearing and the effects of dialect exposure. Ear Hear. 2009;30(5):600–12.

Balance Function of Patients with Common Cavity Deformity

9

Mengya Shen, Xingmei Wei, Xinxing Fu, Ying Kong, and Yongxin Li

As mentioned in Chap. 1, due to the common cavity deformity (CCD) is performed as cochlea and vestibular forming into an ovoid or spherical smooth-walled cystic cavity, in which sensory and supporting cells may be scattered peripherally around the walls of the cavity, and this anatomy characteristic results in severe hearing loss and may accompany with balance dysfunction (Kaga 1999; Livingstone and McPhillips 2011). It is reported that 20% ~70% of the children with hearing loss accompanied with balance and vestibular dysfunction and their vestibular and balance function tests performances were dissatisfied (Said 2014). Researchers have shown that CCD performed poorly in static and dynamic balance skills like dizziness, vertigo, imbalance, gait disorders, and falls. In comparison with their peers, they are at a higher risk for developing gross motor skills and balance strategy (cycling and other items that require a high level of balance control skills) (Melo and Marinho, et al. 2017). In addition, poor balance function may also damage children's psychological behavior, communication skills, and learning interests. For

The original version of this chapter was revised. The correction to this chapter can be found at
https://doi.org/10.1007/978-981-16-8217-9_11

M. Shen (✉) · X. Wei · Y. Li
Department of Otorhinolaryngology Head and Neck Surgery, Beijing Tongren Hospital, Capital Medical University, Beijing, China

Key Laboratory of Otolaryngology Head and Neck Surgery (Capital Medical University), Ministry of Education, Beijing, China

X. Fu · Y. Kong
Key Laboratory of Otolaryngology Head and Neck Surgery (Capital Medical University), Ministry of Education, Beijing, China

Beijing Institute of Otolaryngology, Beijing Tongren Hospital, Capital Medical University, Beijing, China adults, balance disorders affect the quality of life, career, and social performance. Therefore, it is important to evaluate the balance function of sensorineural hearing loss (SNHL). Because early recognition and diagnosis of vestibular dysfunction is important for early treatment and rehabilitation and can improve their quality of life effectively. So do for CCD patients (Walicka-Cuprys and Przygoda, et al. 2014). This chapter describes the assessment of balance function, research progress of evaluation of CCD patients' balance function before and after CI.

9.1   Concept of Balance Function

Balance is a basic need for daily activities and it has a complex and sophisticated mechanism. Balance function is responsible for body posture, gross motor, and response to disturbances, depending primarily on the coordination of visual, vestibular, and somatosensory systems. Balance includes static and dynamic balance (Rine et al. 2000). The static balance is the ability to maintain a stable position in a weight bearing, antigravity posture, and the dynamic balance is the ability to change a position or change position while maintaining stability (Ayanniyi et al. 2014; Cumberworth et al. 2007; Foudriat et al. 1993; Horak et al. 1997).

Balance system develops after birth and becomes mature in a teenager, which relies on the integration of vestibular, visual, and somatosensory systems (Cumberworth et al. 2007). Therefore, the vestibular and balance function tests include open eye tests and closed eye tests. According to development regulation, visual systems play a major role in the development of posture stability in infants, while proprioception and vestibular system may dominate posture control in later lifetime (Foudriat et al. 1993; Horak et al. 1997). Bruininks et al. have previously demonstrated that children with sensorineural hearing loss (SNHL) and bilateral vestibular loss depend more heavily on vision to remain upright than their peers (Deitz et al. 2009) and impairment in any of these systems can cause balance dysfunction.

9.2   Assessment Methods of Balance Function

Balance is maintained by complex interactions between visual, proprioceptive, vestibular, and gross motor systems, and can be divided into dynamic balance tests and static balance function tests (Cushing et al. 2008b; Karakoc and Mujdeci 2021). A brief introduction of the balance function assessment methods and performance in cochlear implantation (CI) patients will be described as follows.

9.2.1   Static Balance Function Tests

Stabilometry is a tool to evaluate static balance function under four kinds of conditions, respectively (Tokita et al. 1981). Condition A: subjects stand on a firm surface with eyes open; Condition B: subjects stand on a firm surface with eyes closed and covered by eyeshades; Condition C: subjects stand on a foam pad with eyes open; Condition D: subjects stand on a foam pad with eyes closed and covered by eyeshades. In 2011, Huang et al. (2011) used stabilometry to assess CI patients' balance function, which needs subject to stand upright over the mark of the platform and keep their body as stable as possible meanwhile the center of gravity (COG) of the subject was recorded for 60s under each of the four above conditions. The results showed that the static balance function of patients with a long-term CI were worse than the normal hearing peers. When both visual and proprioceptive senses were interrupted, the difference between CI and normal hearing groups was largest.

9.2.1.1 Measurement of Standing Balance

The Romberg test was first proposed by Moritz Romberg in 1848 (Apeksha et al. 2021) and it was based on the phenomenon of patients with proprioception dysfunction unable to stand stably while eyes closed. In recent years, some scholars developed this classic test for patients with hearing loss. Participants were required to put their feet together and stand with their eyes open or closed. If subjects occurred obvious shaking or falling with their eyes closed, it indicated the patients with some vestibular dysfunction. The Romberg test can combine with static posturography (SPG) or computerized Dynamic Posturography (CDP) for quantitative evaluation (Bilgec et al. 2021; Karakoc and Mujdeci 2021).

In addition, the single-limb standing test is a clinically commonly used stand-balance measurement tool. It evaluates the posture stability of the static standing position by measuring the time (seconds) when the subject maintains the single-limb standing position (Soori et al. 2019).

9.2.2 Dynamic Balance Function

Gait Balance includes walking test, quick-turn test, tandem Romberg test, Fukuda stepping test, forward bow step test, and Dynamic Gait Index (DGI). It is suitable for patients who can walk by themselves generally (Fukuda 1959; Desmond 2004; Wrisley et al. 2004; Murray et al. 2020; Chow et al. 2021).

Weight-bearing balancing includes standing and squat weight test.

Sensory Organization Test (SOT) is a measurement of dynamic balance and maintaining posture (Casselbrant et al. 2010). It contains three 20-second trials to stand upright on a fixed or movable platform with eyes closed or open. And there are six different sensory testing conditions: (1) eyes open with a fixed platform and surround, (2) eyes closed with a fixed platform and surround, (3) eyes open with a fixed platform and movable surround, (4) eyes open with a movable platform and fixed surround, (5) eyes closed with a movable platform and fixed surround, (6) eyes open with a movable platform and surround (Grove et al. 2021). Each SOT condition emphasizes the ability of equilibrium control and it is the only test for a quantitative assessment of proprioceptive, visual, and vestibular function (Charpiot et al. 2010).

Biodex Balance System (BBS), a balance measurement system (Daud et al. 2021) includes COG movement stability control test and COG rhythm control test which can test postural stability of adults with SNHL and also use for balance training (Dawson et al. 2018).

Tips: To evaluate the degree of cooperation and identify camouflage needs to observe the coincidence of the original curve of each test (repeated more than twice).

9.2.3 Computed Dynamic Posturography

CDP has been used to assess balance in patients with vertigo, but now has been a relatively new test to assess postural stability and fall tendency for vestibular disorders (Oda et al. 1996; Mockford et al. 2011). The test device includes a sensory and a motor component. The sensory component involves a battery of postural control tests which is used to assess the patients' ability to integrate vision, vestibular, and somatosensory senses to maintain balance (Herdman 2013). And motor tests include motor control test (MCT) and adaptation test (Hosseinzadeh et al. 2020).

The test procedure of CDP is as follows. Subject stands or walks on two independent resistance load plates, and the trajectory of COG under different incentive conditions (e.g., vestibular, visual and proprioceptive systems) are recorded by high sensitivity sensors. The tiny movement of COG is expressed in forms of numbers and images after computer processing analysis. The advantage of CDP is that it can relatively separate the information of visual, proprioceptive, and vestibular senses, which is helpful to analyze the abnormal situation of balance dysfunction. CDP can identify patients who are at risk of falling and provide effective and objective treatment planning, and at the same time, it can help understand the pathological physiology of imbalances and contribute to making preventing falls strategies. In addition, the SOT part of CDP is the only quantitative test for assessment of three sensory systems affecting balance (McClay et al. 2002). SOT analysis of CDP can identify the type of sensory abnormality that is responsible for balance impairment (Hosseinzadeh et al. 2020).

9.2.4 Bruininks-Oseretsky Test of Motor Proficiency

Bruininks-Oseretsky Test of Motor Proficiency's (BOTMP) original version was first proposed in 1978 by Bruininks and its second edition was revised in 2005 and called BOT-2 (Bruininks and Bruininks 2005; South and Palilla 2013). BOT-2 aims to assess the athletic proficiency of patients aged 4 years to 21 years and 11 months (Children under 4 years of age can be assessed using motor development scales such as the Gesell Developmental Schedules and the Peabody Motor development Scale) and it is an individually administered test of fine and gross motor skills. BOT-2 intends to evaluate motor performance, specifically fine manual control, manual coordination, body coordination, strength, and agility to assess the overall balance function. BOT-2 has become the most widely used standardized measurement of motor proficiency (Crowe and Horak 1988; Deitz et al. 2007; Charpiot et al. 2010). BOT-2 includes 9 independent tests, of which 4 tests with eyes open and the rest are under close-eyes condition. The BOT-2 raw scores were transformed to an age-scaled score based on normative data (1520 normal developing children). Age-scaled scores range from 1 to 37, and higher scores indicate better static and dynamic balance (Bruininks and Bruininks 2005). Wolter and Gordon et al.'s research in 2021 used BOT-2 to test balance function for children with SNHL and bilateral vestibular loss and found their balance function were worse than normally developing children (Wolter et al. 2021).

9.3   The Balance Function of Inner Ear Malformation and CCD

Inner ear malformations (IEMs) are one reason for vestibular disorders in children and may cause delays in gross motor development (sitting, standing, walking, etc.) (Wiener-Vacher 2008; Sennaroglu and Bajin 2017). As early as 1974, Rapin proposed that congenital vestibular loss can cause delayed gross motor development, such as head control and independent walking (Rapin 1974). Later, in Kaga et al. 1981, Kaga et al. confirmed Rapin's hypothesis by a study of deaf children diagnosed by auditory brainstem response (ABR) and damped rotational chair test (Rapin 1974). Now, many researches have reported the characteristics of congenital disequilibrium in congenital IEM patients, and found that they had weak head stability, retroflexion of the head, and delayed body support under 1-year old, but between 1 and 2 years, because of repaired labyrinthine reflex and acquired gross motor function they would get the ability of independent ambulation (Kimura et al. 2018). Infants and young children mainly rely on the visual system to keep balance, Hosseinzadeh et al. found that with age development, they depended more on vestibular and somatosensory systems, and full maturity of balance function achieved by age of 10 years and motor coordination and adult-like gait pattern matured by 7–10 years old (Hosseinzadeh et al. 2020). In addition, the research also expounded the balance function in 4 CCD patients of 50 SNHL patients who underwent CI by BOT-2 test and there were 22 patients with IEM, among which 4 were CCD, and the results showed balance function of patients without IEMs was better than patients with IEMs.

Rine et al. reported patients with SNHL and bilateral vestibular loss have significantly delayed motor skills and they stand and walk much later than their peers with normal hearing and vestibular function (Rine et al. 2000). The dynamic and static balance performance deficit led to gross motor skill deficiency and balance dysfunction. Because of existence of vestibular nerve deficiency, CCD patients may accompanied with more severe symptoms of the balance dysfunction, such as unstable or vertigo (Maes et al. 2014). In the research of Kaga et al., they found that vestibulo-ocular reflex (VOR) appeared at approximately 3–4 years in CCD patients, and some balance skills and gross motor abilities such as head control and independent walking would delay (Kaga et al. 2019). Until now, most researchers thought the above vestibular development phenomenon of CCD patients is because of the development of proprioception and visual compensation, but not the development of vestibular organ alone (Szymczyk et al. 2012). However, there are no insufficient studies in the postural instability and balance function of patients with CCD.

Butterfeld et al. believe that the balanced state is an integral part of fundamental motor skills, therefore, according to the above analysis, hearing impaired children may present delay in gross motor skills such as catching, kicking, jumping, and hopping, then result in the delay of other motor skills' learning and visual and perceptual developments and the sensory integration function (Rajendran et al. 2013). Childhood is the most important time to learn various skills, and children with hearing impairment accompany by multiple motor, communication, and social disorders and may result in educational, developmental, and social abilities disorders. Thus, early detection of vestibular dysfunction and identifying patients at high risk of vestibular function defects is important for early therapeutic and rehabilitative strategies which can ameliorate functional impairments of CCDs in the future and improve their quality of life.

9.4   Balance Function after Cochlear Implantation

There were studies assessing the effect of hearing with CI on postural control and the results showed that balance function was significantly improved when the implanted device was "ON" (Cushing et al. 2008a; Wolter et al. 2021). Balance function improvement after CIs may be because of electrical stimulation to the vestibular nerve while the auditory nerve was stimulated, especially when the stimulation level was enhanced, the electrical excitability can spread to vestibular areas. Therefore, there was a study found that even under same visual condition, the postural balance after CI was improved (Viljanen et al. 2009).

However, there were studies reporting balance and vestibular function damage after CI surgery and the reason may be because auditory and vestibular receptors have a close relationship, and CI implanted into cochlea can cause balance and vestibular damage and balance problem (surgical trauma during electrode array insertion or electrical stimulation to vestibular nerve), in addition, acute serous labyrinthitis caused by cochlear stoma and foreign body reaction were also possible reasons (Katsiari et al. 2013). It was reported that postoperative vertigo and imbalance occurred in 34% of all CI patients (Steenerson et al. 2001). In patients with CCD, CI may damage the vestibular neurons due to vestibular and cochlear fusion, and aggravate existing balance deficiency, and lead to developmental delays in gross motor activity (Ibrahim et al. 2017).

However, with the improvement of surgical techniques, surgical methods, and modified of electrodes, more CCD patients received CI surgery, for example, transmastoid slotted labyrinthotomy with customized electrode, the incidence and severity of postoperative complications like facial nerve injury, insertion into the internal auditory canal and cerebral spinal fluid leakage were reduced and the postoperative effect was gradually improved (Al-Mahboob et al. 2021).

In addition, Vestibular Rehabilitation (VR) treatment plans can help patients to get early compensation, and then reduce the symptoms of imbalance, and have a positive impact on the life quality of patients (Bonucci et al. 2008; Saki et al. 2020). General balance rehabilitation can strengthen the proprioceptive and visual systems' input and output and VR programs can combine specific head movements with gaze stability exercises to reduce dizziness and imbalance (Nafaji et al. 2021). The common goal of VR was to improve CI users' quality of life by enabling the patient to proceed with auditory and speech rehabilitation and maintain balance. In 2017, there was a report about VR for a 54-year-old patient who underwent CI, and after 14 sessions last over 4 months' static and dynamic standing balance exercises with varied foot positions and support bases. The exercise methods integrated with alternating optokinetic stimulation, visual and vocal stimulation, and the exercise environments include walking indoors and outdoors, on stairs, busy streets, and shopping malls (Zur et al. 2017). Shah et al. reported a study for 10 hearing impaired patients aged 6–12 years old using balance training, hand–eye coordination, visual–motor coordination, and overall coordination training, and the training schedule was 10 min per day, 3 days per week, and lasted for 12 weeks and the research found that these exercises could improve the overall motor skills and posture control for hearing impaired patients (Shah et al. 2013). But there was no report about VR for children CCD patients, which needs further research.

We suggest that in future studies, CCD patients should be participated to reveal the effect of balance training for CI results. And balance function should be combined with vestibular function to provide more accurate and complete assessment data. Contents about the progress of vestibular function in CI patients will be introduced in the next chapter.

9.5 Conclusion

In conclusion, the balance function test mainly includes static balance function test, dynamic evaluation function test, CDP and BOT-2. At present, studies have found that the balance function of CCD patients was worse than that of normal patients, but some studies showed that the balance function after CI can be significantly improved. At last, it is suggested that because balance function is an important part of physical development, the perfect pre- and postoperative evaluation and rehabilitation systems are of great significance for the improvement of patient's life quality.

References

Al-Mahboob A, Alhabib SF, et al. Cochlear implantation in common cavity deformity: a systematic review. Eur Arch Otorhinolaryngol. 2021;

Apeksha K, Singh S, et al. Balance assessment of children with sensorineural hearing loss. Ind J Otolaryngol Head Neck Surg. 2021;73(1):12–7.

Ayanniyi O, Adepoju FA, et al. Static and dynamic balance in school children with and without hearing impairment. Journal of Experimental & Integrative Medicine. 2014;4(4):245–8.

Beth A, Foudriat Richard P, Di Fabio John H, Anderson. Sensory organization of balance responses in children 3–6 years of age: a normative study with diagnostic implications. International Journal of Pediatric Otorhinolaryngology. 1993;27(3):255–71. 10.1016/0165-5876(93)90231-Q.

Bilgec MD, Erdogmus KN, et al. Evaluation of the vestibulocochlear system in patients with Pseudoexfoliation syndrome. Turk J Ophthalmol. 2021;51(3):156–60.

Bonucci AS, Costa FO, et al. Vestibular function in cochlear implant users. Braz J Otorhinolaryngol. 2008;74(2):273–8.

Bruininks BD, Bruininks RH. Bruininks-Oseretsky Test of Motor Proficiency, 2nd edition (BOT-2). 2005.

Casselbrant ML, Mandel EM, et al. Longitudinal posturography and rotational testing in children three to nine years of age: normative data. Otolaryngol Head Neck Surg. 2010;142(5):708–14.

Cumberworth NN, Patel W, Rogers GS, Kenyon VL. The maturation of balance in children. The Journal of Laryngology & Otology. 2007;121(5):449–54. https://doi.org/10.1017/S0022215106004051.

Charpiot A, Tringali S, et al. Vestibulo-ocular reflex and balance maturation in healthy children aged from six to twelve years. Audiol Neurootol. 2010;15(4):203–10.

Chow MR, Ayiotis AI, et al. Posture, gait, quality of life, and hearing with a vestibular implant. N Engl J Med. 2021;384(6):521–32.

Crowe TK, Horak FB. Motor proficiency associated with vestibular deficits in children with hearing impairments. Phys Ther. 1988;68(10):1493–9.

Cushing SL, Chia R, et al. A test of static and dynamic balance function in children with cochlear implants: the vestibular olympics. Arch Otolaryngol Head Neck Surg. 2008a;134(1):34–8.

Cushing SL, Papsin BC, et al. Evidence of vestibular and balance dysfunction in children with profound sensorineural hearing loss using cochlear implants. Laryngoscope. 2008b;118(10):1814–23.

Daud S, Rahman MU, et al. Effect of balance training with Biodex balance system to improve balance in patients with diabetic neuropathy: a quasi experimental study. Pak J Med Sci. 2021;37(2):389–92.

Dawson N, Dzurino D, et al. Examining the reliability, correlation, and validity of commonly used assessment tools to measure balance. Health Sci Rep. 2018;1(12):e98.

Deitz JC, Kartin D, et al. Review of the Bruininks-Oseretsky test of motor proficiency, second edition (BOT-2). Phys Occup Ther Pediatr. 2007;27(4):87–102.

Deitz JC, Kartin D, et al. Review of the Bruininks-Oseretsky test of motor proficiency, second edition (BOT-2). Phys Occup Ther Pediatr. 2009;

Desmond A. Vestibular function: evaluation and treatment, vestibular function: evaluation and treatment. 2004.

Fay B, Horak Sharon M, Henry Anne, Shumway-Cook. Postural Perturbations: New Insights for Treatment of Balance Disorders. Physical Therapy. 1997;77(5):517–33. 10.1093/ptj/77.5.517.

Fukuda T. The stepping test: two phases of the labyrinthine reflex. Acta Otolaryngol. 1959;50(2):95–108.

Grove CR, Whitney SL, et al. Effect of repetitive Administration of a Next-generation Sensory Organization Test in adults with and without vestibular dysfunction. Otol Neurotol. 2021;42(3):e363–70.

Herdman SJ. Vestibular rehabilitation. Curr Opin Neurol. 2013;26(1):96–101.

Hosseinzadeh F, Asghari A, et al. Balance function after cochlear implant and inner ear anomaly: comparison of dynamic posturography. Laryngoscope Investig Otolaryngol. 2020;5(3):529–35.

Huang MW, Hsu CJ, et al. Static balance function in children with cochlear implants. Int J Pediatr Otorhinolaryngol. 2011;75(5):700–3.

Ibrahim I, Da SS, et al. Effect of cochlear implant surgery on vestibular function: meta-analysis study. J Otolaryngol Head Neck Surg. 2017;46(1):44.

Kaga K. Vestibular compensation in infants and children with congenital and acquired vestibular loss in both ears. Int J Pediatr Otorhinolaryngol. 1999;49(3):215–24.

Kaga K, Suzuki JI, et al. Influence of labyrinthine hypoactivity on gross motor development of infants. Ann N Y Acad Sci. 1981;374:412–20.

Kaga K, Kimura Y, et al. Development of vestibular ocular reflex and gross motor function in infants with common cavity deformity as a type of inner ear malformation. Acta Otolaryngol. 2019:1–6.

Karakoc K, Mujdeci B. Evaluation of balance in children with sensorineural hearing loss according to age. Am J Otolaryngol. 2021;42(1):102830.

Katsiari E, Balatsouras DG, et al. Influence of cochlear implantation on the vestibular function. Eur Arch Otorhinolaryngol. 2013;270(2):489–95.

Kimura Y, Masuda T, et al. Vestibular function and gross motor development in 195 children with congenital hearing loss-assessment of inner ear malformations. Otol Neurotol. 2018;39(2):196–205.

Livingstone N, McPhillips M. Motor skill deficits in children with partial hearing. Dev Med Child Neurol. 2011;53(9):836–42.

Maes L, De Kegel A, et al. Association between vestibular function and motor performance in hearing-impaired children. Otol Neurotol. 2014;35(10):e343–7.

McClay JE, Tandy R, et al. Major and minor temporal bone abnormalities in children with and without congenital sensorineural hearing loss. Arch Otolaryngol Head Neck Surg. 2002;128(6):664–71.

Melo RS, Marinho S, et al. Static and dynamic balance of children and adolescents with sensorineural hearing loss. Einstein (Sao Paulo). 2017;15(3):262–8.

Mockford KA, Mazari FA, et al. Computerized dynamic posturography in the objective assessment of balance in patients with intermittent claudication. Ann Vasc Surg. 2011;25(2):182–90.

Murray D, Viani L, et al. Balance, gait and dizziness in adult cochlear implant users: a cross sectional study. Cochlear Implants Int. 2020;21(1):46–52.

Nafaji S, Abshirini H, et al. Comparison of vestibular rehabilitation on balance function in cochlear implant recipients. Int Tinnitus J. 2021;25(1):10–2.

Oda D, Ganança CF, et al. Computerized dynamic posturography in the assessment of body balance in individuals with vestibular dysfunction. Anaesthesia. 1996;51(51):611–1.

Rajendran V, Roy FG, et al. Effect of exercise intervention on vestibular related impairments in hearing-impaired children. Alexandria Journal of Medicine. 2013;49(1):7–12.

Rapin I. Hypoactive labyrinths and motor development. Clin Pediatr (Phila). 1974;13(11):922–3, 926–9, 934–7.

Rine RM, Cornwall G, et al. Evidence of progressive delay of motor development in children with sensorineural hearing loss and concurrent vestibular dysfunction. Percept Mot Skills. 2000;90(3 Pt 2):1101–12.

Said E. Vestibular assessment in children with sensorineural hearing loss using both electronystagmography and vestibular-evoked myogenic potential. English World-Wide. 2014;30(1):333.

Saki N, Abshirini H, et al. Investigating the effects of vestibular rehabilitation on balance function in Cochlear implant recipients. Int Tinnitus J. 2020;24(1):36–9.

Sennaroglu L, Bajin MD. Classification and current Management of Inner ear Malformations. Balkan Med J. 2017;34(5):397–411.

Shah J, Rao K, et al. Effect of motor control program in improving gross motor function and postural control in children with sensorineural hearing loss-a pilot study. Pediatr Therapeut S. 2013;03(1)

Soori Z, Heyrani A, et al. Exercise effects on motor skills in hearing-impaired children. Sport Sciences for Health. 2019;4

South M, Palilla J. Bruininks-Oseretsky test of motor proficiency, bruininks-oseretsky test of motor proficiency. 2013.

Steenerson RL, Cronin GW, et al. Vertigo after cochlear implantation. Otol Neurotol. 2001;22(6):842–3.

Szymczyk D, Druzbicki M, et al. Balance and postural stability in football players with hearing impairment. 2012.

Tokita T, Maeda M, et al. The role of the labyrinth in standing posture regulation. Acta Otolaryngol. 1981;91(5–6):521–7.

Viljanen A, Kaprio J, et al. Hearing as a predictor of falls and postural balance in older female twins. J Gerontol A Biol Sci Med Sci. 2009;64(2):312–7.

Walicka-Cuprys K, Przygoda L, et al. Balance assessment in hearing-impaired children. Res Dev Disabil. 2014;35(11):2728–34.

Wiener-Vacher SR. Vestibular disorders in children. Int J Audiol. 2008;47(9):578–83.

Wolter NE, Gordon KA, et al. Impact of the sensory environment on balance in children with bilateral cochleovestibular loss. Hear Res. 2021;400:108134.

Wrisley DM, Marchetti GF, et al. Reliability, internal consistency, and validity of data obtained with the functional gait assessment. Phys Ther. 2004;84(10):906–18.

Zur O, Ben-Rubi SH, et al. Balance versus hearing after cochlear implant in an adult. BMJ Case Rep. 2017;2017

Vestibular Function of Patient with Common Cavity Deformity

10

Xingmei Wei, Jingyuan Chen, Ying Kong, Yongxin Li, and Xinxing Fu

The vestibule organs were developed from the dorsal pouch of otic vesicle at 4–5 weeks gestation (WG) (Streeter 1906) and matured during 4–20 WG, which are related to development of cochlea. Patients with inner ear malformation may be accompanied with vestibular dysfunction, and there were researches reported that in some deaf children, they occurred vestibular loss and gross motor development delay (Rapin and I. 1974) and the rate can achieve 60% (Jacot et al. 2009). Especially for patients with common cavity deformity (CCD), the vestibule and cochlear are fused together and the vestibular neurons may be limited. What is more, CCD often accompanied with cochlear nerve deficiency (CND), which may have vestibular sensory cells abnormalities (Kaga et al. 2008). Therefore, the necessity of vestibular assessment for cochlear implantation (CI) in children is increasingly urgent. Some scholars suggested vestibular assessment must be routinely performed in each reference CI center (Coudert et al. 2017). In this chapter, we will introduce the vestibular assessment methods and the vestibular function variation before and after CI surgery, especially in CCD patients.

X. Wei (✉) · J. Chen · Y. Li
Department of Otorhinolaryngology Head and Neck Surgery, Beijing Tongren Hospital, Capital Medical University, Beijing, China

Key Laboratory of Otolaryngology Head and Neck Surgery (Capital Medical University), Ministry of Education, Beijing, China

Y. Kong · X. Fu
Key Laboratory of Otolaryngology Head and Neck Surgery (Capital Medical University), Ministry of Education, Beijing, China

Beijing Institute of Otolaryngology, Beijing Tongren Hospital, Capital Medical University, Beijing, China

© The Author(s), under exclusive license to Springer Nature Singapore Pte Ltd. 2022
Y. Li (ed.), *Cochlear Implantation for Common Cavity Deformity*,
https://doi.org/10.1007/978-981-16-8217-9_10

10.1   Vestibular Assessment Methods

The vestibular consists of semicircular canals and otolith, and the test for semicircular canals mainly include caloric test, rotatory test, and video head impulse test (vHIT), and the test for otolith mainly includes vestibular evoked myogenic potential (VEMP) test (Fig. 10.1). What is more, there are questionnaires about evaluating vestibular function, such as dizziness handicap inventory (DHI) and pediatric vestibular symptom questionnaire (PVSQ).

10.1.1 The Caloric Test

The caloric test evaluates the responses of the two lateral semicircular canals at low frequencies (about 0.003 Hz) and is not suitable for little children (Jongkees 1948). There were researches comparing the caloric test results before and after CI surgery and finding a decrease after surgery. For example, Chen et al. (2016) found a rate of 34.5% increase of semicircular canals function injury four weeks after CI in a study of 34 patients. Enticott et al. (2006) did an analysis for 46 patients and found that in 32% patients occurred semicircular canals injury 1 week after CI surgery according to caloric test. However, there was also report that found 8 of 49 patients observed vestibular improvement evaluated by caloric test and thought the reason may be because of electronic stimulation for labyrinth (Ribári et al. 1999).

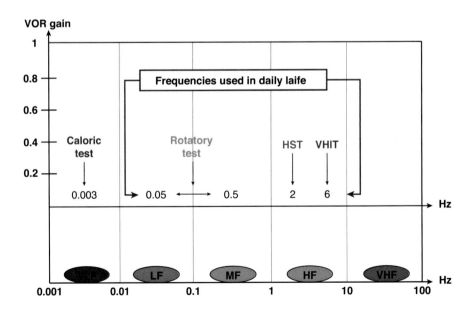

Fig. 10.1 The frequency range of vestibular receptors. *VLF* very low frequency, *LF* low frequency, *MF* medium frequency, *HF* high frequency, *VHF* very high frequency, *HST* Head Shaking Test, *VHIT* Video Head Impulse Test (reproduced with permission from Coudert et al. 2017)

10.1.2 The Rotatory Test

The rotatory test evaluates the function of the two lateral semicircular canals to low and medium frequency stimulations which also need the patients are over 5–6 years old (Maes et al. 2007) and its response is recorded by vestibulo–ocular reflex. If there is vestibular deficiency, the reflex is abolished or diminished.

10.1.3 The Video Head Impulse Test

The vHIT assesses the function of the six semicircular canals for high frequency stimulation, because it does not require wearing goggles, it is suitable for little children. And researches showed that the change after CI surgery of VHIT test was much smaller than caloric test and researchers considered that the high frequency area of the semicircular canal damaged only when the low frequency damage was severe (Migliaccio et al. 2005; Melvin et al. 2009; Beynon et al. 2010; Jutila et al. 2013). For example, Jutila et al. (2013) found that only in 10% of 44 patients after CI surgery occurred change of HIT and Migliaccio et al. (2005) reported that 1 of 11 patients displayed injury of high frequency vestibulo–ocular reflex. The results showed CI surgery affected the function of type I vestibular hair cell rarely.

10.1.4 The Vestibular Evoked Myogenic Potential Test

VEMP evaluates the otolith function and it includes cervical-VEMP (c-VEMP) and ocular-VEMP (o-VEMP). The c-VEMP is feasible for little children and infants, even as little as 2 months of age (Wiener-Vacher 2004; Kelsch et al. 2006). VEMP is the most commonly used test on the evaluation of vestibular function in CI patients and the possible reasons may be because the sacculus is close to the cochlea and the sacculus injury risk of CI surgery is bigger than semicircular canals, it is necessary to evaluate the functional status of the sacculus. In addition, meta-analysis showed that VEMPs were more sensitive than other vestibular function tests (Moreau et al. 2017) and the results revealed a sensitivity of 0.21 (CI 95% 0.08–0.40) for the caloric tests, of 0.32 (CI 95% 0.15–0.54) for the c-VEMP. Researches also showed that for severe deafness children, the VEMPs were easier to be abnormal than children with normal hearing and the difference was significant (Zhou et al. 2009; Singh et al. 2012). There were reports founding that for patients with normal vestibular function before surgery, about 60–86% occurred VEMP abolished or diminished after CI (Krause et al. 2009; Katsiari et al. 2013).

10.1.5 The Dizziness Handicap Inventory

The DHI is popularly used in clinical for patients' subjective impression about their vestibular and balance function and consists of 25 items, 9 of which were related to emotion (E), 9 to function (F), and 7 to physical (P) (Tamber et al. 2009). There are researches recommending to combine subjective and objective assessments together to evaluate vestibular function (Guan et al. 2021; Weinmann et al. 2021). Muhammed et al. used DHI to evaluate 42 patients' vestibular function before and after CI surgery and found DHI score increase in 12 of 42 patients (vestibular function impairment) (Muhammed et al. 2018). However, a meta-analysis about 25 patients came to a different conclusion and the results showed DHI scores were not significantly affected after CI surgery (Ibrahim et al. 2017).

10.1.6 The Pediatric Vestibular Symptom Questionnaire

The PVSQ can evaluate the severity of vestibular symptoms (dizziness, instability) in children aged 6–17 years old and contains 10 multiple choice questions and 1 subjective essay question (Godfrey et al. 2016). Guan et al. (2021) reported that PVSQ scores between pre- and post-implantation for unilateral CI showed no significant difference, but in children with bilateral CI, PVSQ scores increased significantly 3 days after surgery and significantly decreased after 30 days, and they considered the changes may be due to the acute reaction to anesthesia or middle/inner ear trauma during surgery.

10.2 Vestibular Function Pre- and Post-Cochlear Implantation Surgery

From the above, vHIT for high frequencies and c-VEMP for otolith function are more usually used for children with cochlear implantation (CI). Certainly, most studies used multiple vestibular function assessment methods and there have been studies about vestibular function pre- and post-CI surgery (Craig et al. 2004; Jacot et al. 2009; Licameli et al. 2010; Huang et al. 2011; Psillas et al. 2014; Kegel et al. 2015; Ajalloueyan et al. 2017; West et al. 2020) and found that about 50% of pediatric CI candidates have vestibular deficits and 51% of implants induce vestibular function modifications (Jacot et al. 2009) and vestibular hypofunction of different vestibular organs varies (West et al. 2020). The vestibular function after CI surgery may be impaired, unchanged, or improved.

Many literatures found that the vestibular function impaired after CI surgery and further analysis indicated that c-VEMPs were the most often impaired, followed by the caloric test, and the HIT were the most often conserved (Abouzayd et al. 2016; Koyama et al. 2021). The reason may be because saccule is adjacent to cochlea. Handzel et al. (2006) explored 19 temporal bone and found that 59% (10/17) CI temporal bone occurred cochlear hydrops, among which 80% (8/10) was saccule collapse. Salvinelli et al. (1999) also found the saccule injured mostly by 4 temporal bone implanted CI 10 years from histopathological level. Other factors such as labyrinthitis, electrode insertion, electrical stimulation, drill damage, fibrosis, and ossification may also cause vestibular function impairment (Ito 1998; Hui-Chi et al. 2002). And the surgical approach also affected the vestibular function, Todt et al.

found a significant difference of postoperative VEMP responses (50% vs 13%) between cochleostomy and round window approaches (Todt et al. 2008). In addition, Koyama et al. (2021) found that the perimodiolar electrodes affected caloric test results greater than straight electrodes which indicated electrodes type is another factor that influences vestibular function. Some researchers showed that CI surgery impaired vestibular function of the non-implanted side (Bonucci et al. 2008; Katsiari et al. 2013). Katsiari et al. (2013) by the caloric test showed that the semicircular canal function on the non-implanted side changed from normal before surgery to paresthesia after surgery. Bonucci et al. (2008) also found some patients with CI had bilateral vestibular function decline. Vibert et al. 2001 also reported similar findings, and suggested that the absence of vestibular response in the non-implanted side might be related to the development of bilateral progressive inner ear disease. Katsiari et al. (2013) believed that the decreased vestibular function on the non-implanted side might be due to the electrode insertion to the scala tympani which influences the signal input from the vestibular to the brain or the formation of a complex vestibular response on the non-implanted side. Another possible reason was that the repair function of vestibular injuries in individual patients may decline over time. In addition, bilateral implantation may increase the risk of vestibular loss, for example, Wagner et al. (2010) evaluated 20 cases with DHI and found that after the second implantation, the DHI scores increased significantly compared with the first implantation.

However, there was also a prospective cohort study about 27 children 1–4 years old whose vestibular function was evaluated by caloric test, HIT, and VEMP before and after CI surgery, and they found no significant change (Ajalloueyan et al. 2017). They considered the differences coming from age and this study's postoperative tests were performed before activating CI prostheses. Vibert et al. (2001) also found the otolithic function of all 6 CI patients was preserved after surgery.

In addition, there were a few researches that even found vestibular function improvement after CI surgery (Ribári et al. 1999; Craig et al. 2004; Bonucci et al. 2008; Katsiari et al. 2013). Bonucci et al. (2008) found that 13% patients showed no vestibular disorder after CI, 5% showed worsening and 13% showed an improvement and they considered it was caused by electric stimulation of labyrinth. Bonucci et al. (2008) observed the vestibular function of 38 patients with CI by electronystagmus, and the results showed that 13% of the patients had vestibular function improvement after implantation, and the authors thought this may be related to vestibular compensation and stimulation current. Katsiari et al. (2013) also reported a case of transient improvement of horizontal semicircular canal function on the implanted side after CI surgery by the caloric test but returned to normal 1 month after surgery, and back to the preoperative state 6 months after surgery. Katsiari et al. (2013) thought that the initial improvement in vestibular function was due to a temporary readjustment of the vestibular system.

The results above indicated us a rigorous clinical examination combined with a vestibular analysis must be conducted and the vestibular evaluation can help distinguish between the vestibular impairment linked to deafness and those induced by

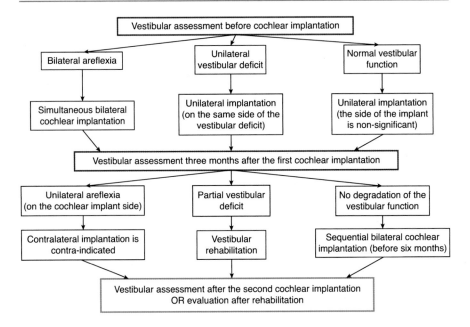

Fig. 10.2 Cochlear implantation scheduling based on the vestibular assessment (reproduced with permission from Coudert et al. 2017)

the CI and further guides the choice of CI side, especially for patients with bilateral CI. Appropriate counseling and management must be provided if vestibular damage occurs postoperatively. Even if these children currently do not have vestibular symptoms, it is still necessary to understand their vestibular functioning status, because the CI induced vestibular impairment will be more difficult to recover in the future, that is, as they get older or have other causes of vestibular impairment (Licameli et al. 2010). The vestibular assessment schedule before and after CI surgery is shown in Fig. 10.2.

10.3 Vestibular Function of Common Cavity Deformity

As for vestibular assessment for CCD patients, it was first reported in 2018 by Kaga et al. (2019). They tested eight CCD infants with damped rotational chair test regularly and also compared their head control and independent walking with normal infants and found that the CCD infants' vestibular ocular reflex was not present around the first year but appeared after three or 4 years and head control and independent walking were delayed but eventually acquired. They also put forward two hypotheses to explain the results: (1) the vestibular sensory cells may become mature by stimulation of endolymphatic flow, (2) the central vestibular compensating mechanism could help gross motor and balance function development (Kaga

2014). Our center also found the vestibular function test for CCD patients usually cannot be elicited.

About the vestibular function of CCD patients after CI surgery, in 2001, Sennaroglu et al. (2001) reported a CCD patient occurred nystagmus when the implant was stimulated and they put forward a concept of common vestibulocochlear nerve (CVN), because the MRI showed CVN entered the cavity without dividing into cochlear and vestibular branches, and the patient occurred nystagmus probably due to direct stimulation of the vestibular component of the CVN. In our center, we also observed some CCD patients performed slightly tilting forth and back during their cochlear programming. We retrospectively analysed 25 cases (27 ears), four patients displayed slightly tilting forth and back due to vestibular nerve stimulation and the symptoms were caused by no.4, no. 5, no.7 and no. 4 to 6 electrodes, respectively. Then after adjusting the stimulation current the tilting phenomenon disappeared. In 2006, Jin et al. (2006) reported VEMP results of 12 patients under the three condition: before CI surgery, after CI surgery with CI off and after CI surgery with CI on, and there was one CCD patient, his results were that when before CI surgery and after CI surgery with CI off, the VEMPs were absent, and when CI on, VEMPs were present, which further indicated that CI may stimulate vestibular nerve in CCD patients. In that research, patients with other inner ear malformation, such as incomplete partition and CND also demonstrated the same results. In 2017, Kaga and Kimitaka (2017) in their book also described 7 cases' VEMP results and showed they all have VEMP response with CI on. They included 2 CCD, 2 incomplete partition type I, 1 incomplete partition type II, and 1 CND patient. There was some patients showed no VEMPs before CI, but showed VEMPs when CI on, they considered this phenomenon indicated that the sensory cells of saccule may be absent, but the inferior vestibular neurons may by present, especially in CCD patients (Kaga 2014). The vestibular function of CCD patients and the development after CI surgery are desired to be discovered by a large sample size study and long-time follow-up. In addition, for patients with bilateral vestibular asymmetry, researchers considered that they are at a high risk of permanent vestibular disease. Therefore, adequate preoperative evaluation of vestibular function before CI can provide presence or absence of vestibular function and help surgeon selecting suitable side to avoid bilateral vestibular function loss, and experience showed that the side with poor vestibular balance function should be selected for surgery if there is no significant difference in bilateral auditory conditions (Bittar et al. 2017). It is also necessary to evaluate vestibular function after CI to seek for vestibular rehabilitation (VR) treatment plans (see Chap. 9).

10.4 Conclusion

All above, there are several vestibular function assessment methods and in order to evaluate a patient's vestibular function comprehensively, combining multiple assessment methods together is recommended. The vestibular function may impair after CI surgery, but for some patients, the vestibular function improved. However, for patients with CCD, due to its special anatomy, the vestibular function maybe inborn different with others and normal value of varied examination could be different. The vestibular function pre- and post-CI surgery maybe different with other candidates, and the vestibular nerve could be stimulated by electrodes.

References

Abouzayd M, Smith PF, et al. What vestibular tests to choose in symptomatic patients after a cochlear implant? A systematic review and meta-analysis. Arch Klin Exp Ohren Nasen Kehlkopfheilkd. 2016;274(1):1–11.

Ajalloueyan M, Saeedi M, et al. The effects of cochlear implantation on vestibular function in 1–4 years old children. Int J Pediatr Otorhinolaryngol. 2017;94:100.

Beynon, Jani, et al. A clinical evaluation of head impulse testing. Clin Otolaryngol Allied Sci. 2010;23(2):117–22.

Bittar R, Sato ES, et al. Preoperative vestibular assessment protocol of cochlear implant surgery: an analytical descriptive study. Braz J Otorhinolaryngol. 2017;83(5):530–5.

Bonucci AS, Costa FO, et al. Vestibular function in cochlear implant users. Braz J Otorhinolaryngol. 2008;74(2):273–8.

Chen X, Chen X, et al. Influence of cochlear implantation on vestibular function. Acta Otolaryngol. 2016;655

Coudert A, Van HT, et al. Vestibular assessment in Cochlear implanted children: how to do? When to do? A review of literature. Curr Otorhinolaryngol Rep. 2017;5(4):259–67.

Craig and A., et al. Vestibular effects of cochlear implantation. Laryngoscope. 2004.

Enticott JC, Tari S, et al. Cochlear implant and vestibular function. Otol Neurotol. 2006;27(6):824–30.

Godfrey, Emma, et al. The Pediatric vestibular symptom questionnaire: a validation study. J Pediatr. 2016;168:171–7.

Guan R, Wang Y, et al. Vestibular function in children and adults before and after unilateral or sequential bilateral Cochlear implantation. Front Neurol. 2021;12:675502.

Handzel O, Burgess BJ, et al. Histopathology of the peripheral vestibular system after Cochlear implantation in the human. Otol Neurotol. 2006;27(1):57–64.

Huang MW, Hsu CJ, et al. Static balance function in children with cochlear implants. Int J Pediatr Otorhinolaryngol. 2011;75(5):700–3.

Hui-Chi, Tien, et al. Histopathologic changes in the vestibule after cochlear implantation. Otolaryngol Head Neck Surg. 2002;127(4):260–4.

Ibrahim I, Silva S, et al. Effect of cochlear implant surgery on vestibular function: meta-analysis study. J Otolaryngol Head Neck Surg. 2017;46(1):44.

Ito J. Influence of the multichannel cochlear implant on vestibular function. Otolaryngol Head Neck Surg. 1998;118(6):900.

Jacot E, Van Den Abbeele T, et al. Vestibular impairments pre- and post-cochlear implant in children. Int J Pediatr Otorhinolaryngol. 2009;73(2):209–17.

Jin Y, Nakamura M, et al. Vestibular-evoked myogenic potentials in cochlear implant children. Acta Otolaryngol. 2006;126(2):164–9.

Jongkees L. VALUE OF THE CALORIC TEST OF THE LABYRINTH. Arch Otolaryngol Head Neck Surg. 1948;48(4):402–17.

Jutila T, Aalto H, et al. Cochlear implantation rarely alters horizontal vestibulo-ocular reflex in motorized head impulse test. Otol Neurotol. 2013;34(1):48–52.

Kaga K. Vertigo and balance disorders in children. Springer; 2014.

Kaga and Kimitaka. Cochlear implantation in children with inner ear malformation and Cochlear nerve deficiency. Singapore: Springer; 2017.

Kaga K, Shinjo Y, et al. Vestibular failure in children with congenital deafness. Int J Audiol. 2008;47(9):590–9.

Kaga K, Suzuki JI, et al. INFLUENCE OF LABYRINTHINE HYPOACTIVITY ON GROSS MOTOR DEVELOPMENT OF INFANTS. Ann N Y Acad Sci. 2010;374:412–20. (Vestibular and Oculomotor Physiology: International Meeting of the Barany Society)

Kaga K, Kimura Y, et al. Development of vestibular ocular reflex and gross motor function in infants with common cavity deformity as a type of inner ear malformation. Acta Otolaryngol. 2019:1–6.

Katsiari E, Balatsouras DG, et al. Influence of cochlear implantation on the vestibular function. Eur Arch Otorhinolaryngol. 2013;270(2):489–95.

Kegel AD, Maes L, et al. Examining the impact of Cochlear implantation on the early gross motor development of children with a hearing loss. Ear & Hearing. 2015;36(3):e113.

Kelsch TA, Schaefer LA, et al. Vestibular evoked myogenic potentials in young children: test parameters and normative data. Laryngoscope. 2006;166(6):895–900.

Koyama H, Kashio A, et al. Alteration of vestibular function in Pediatric Cochlear implant recipients. Front Neurol. 2021;12:661302.

Krause E, Louza JP, et al. Incidence and quality of vertigo symptoms after cochlear implantation. J Laryngol Otol. 2009;123(3):278–82.

Licameli G, Zhou G, et al. Disturbance of vestibular function attributable to cochlear implantation in children. Laryngoscope. 2010;119(4):740–5.

Maes L, Vinck BM, et al. Evaluation of the rotatory vestibular test: exploration of stimulus parameters. B-ENT. 2007;3(3):119.

Melvin TAN, Santina CD, et al. The effects of Cochlear implantation on vestibular function. Otol Neurotol. 2009;30(2):P60–0.

Migliaccio AA, Santina C, et al. "the vestibulo-ocular reflex response to head impulses rarely decreases after cochlear implantation." otology & neurotology : official publication of the American Otological Society, American Neurotology Society [and] European academy of. Otol Neurotol. 2005;26(4):655.

Moreau and Sylvain, et al. What vestibular tests to choose in symptomatic patients after a cochlear implant? A systematic review and meta-analysis. Eur Arch Otorhinolaryngol Suppl. 2017;274(1):53–63.

Muhammed D, Ulku T, et al. How does cochlear implantation affect five vestibular end-organ functions and dizziness? Auris Nasus Larynx. 2018;46 https://doi.org/10.1016/j.anl.2018.07.004.

Psillas G, Pavlidou A, et al. Vestibular evoked myogenic potentials in children after cochlear implantation. Auris Nasus Larynx. 2014;41(5):432–5.

Rapin and I. Hypoactive labyrinths and motor development. Clin Pediatr. 1974;13(11):922–37.

Ribári O, Küstel M, et al. Cochlear implantation influences contralateral hearing and vestibular responsiveness. Acta Otolaryngol. 1999;119(2):225–8.

Salvinelli F, Trivelli M, et al. Cochlear implant. Histopathological guide to indications and contraindications: a post mortem study on temporal bones. Eur Rev Med Pharmacol Sci. 1999;3(5):217–20.

Sennaroglu L, Gursel B, et al. Vestibular stimulation after cochlear implantation in common cavity deformity. Otolaryngol Head Neck Surg. 2001;125(4):408–10.

Singh S, Gupta RK, et al. Vestibular evoked myogenic potentials in children with sensorineural hearing loss. Int J Pediatr Otorhinolaryngol. 2012;76(9)

Streeter GL. On the development of the membranous labyrinth and the acoustic and facial nerves in the human embryo. Am J Anat. 1906;6(1):139–65.

Tamber AL, Wilhelmsen KT, et al. Measurement properties of the dizziness handicap inventory by cross-sectional and longitudinal designs. Health Q Life Outcomes. 2009;7(1):101–1.

Todt I, Basta D, et al. Does the surgical approach in cochlear implantation influence the occurrence of postoperative vertigo? Otolaryngol Head Neck Surg. 2008;138(1):8–12.

Vibert, Usler RH, et al. Vestibular function in patients with cochlear implantation. Acta Otolaryngol. 2001;121(545):29–34.

Wagner JH, Basta D, et al. Vestibular and taste disorders after bilateral cochlear implantation. Eur Arch Otorhinolaryngol. 2010;267(12):1849–54.

Weinmann C, Baumann U, et al. Vertigo associated with Cochlear implant surgery: correlation with vertigo diagnostic result, electrode carrier, and insertion angle. Front Neurol. 2021;12

West N, Tian L, et al. Objective vestibular test battery and patient reported outcomes in cochlear implant recipients. Otol Neurotol publish ahead of print. 2020.

Wiener-Vacher SR. Vertigo in children. Archives De Pédiatrie Organe Officiel De La Sociéte Franaise De Pédiatrie. 2004;11(12):1542–5.

Zhou G, Kenna MA, et al. Assessment of saccular function in children with sensorineural hearing loss. Arch Otolaryngol Head Neck Surg. 2009;135(1):40–4.

Correction to: Cochlear Implantation for Common Cavity Deformity

Yongxin Li

Correction to:
The book in: Y. Li (ed.), Cochlear Implantation for Common Cavity Deformity,
https://doi.org/10.1007/978-981-16-8217-9

The book was inadvertently published with errors and the following corrections need to be updated:

Correction to:
Chapter 1 in: Y. Li (ed.), Cochlear Implantation for Common Cavity Deformity,
https://doi.org/10.1007/978-981-16-8217-9_1

Reference citation in line 2 of page 7 was published with incorrect caption. This has now been corrected to [right] from [left].

Chapter 3 in: Y. Li (ed.), Cochlear Implantation for Common Cavity Deformity,
https://doi.org/10.1007/978-981-16-8217-9_3

Reference citation in line 22 of page 27 was published with incorrect caption. This has now been corrected to [3.5a] from [3.4a].

Reference citation in line 5 of page 29 was published with incorrect caption. This has now been corrected to [loop] from [look].

Reference citation of fig 3.5 of page 28 was published with incorrect caption.

The updated online version of this chapter can be found at
https://doi.org/10.1007/978-981-16-8217-9_1
https://doi.org/10.1007/978-981-16-8217-9_3
https://doi.org/10.1007/978-981-16-8217-9_4
https://doi.org/10.1007/978-981-16-8217-9_5
https://doi.org/10.1007/978-981-16-8217-9_7
https://doi.org/10.1007/978-981-16-8217-9_9

Please add "(reproduced with permission from Young et al. 2012)" after "(a) Sample 1 of CC shows two prominent dots in the c/s of IAC";

Reference citation of fig 3.9 and 3.10 of page 39 was published with incorrect caption.
Please add "(reproduced with permission from Wei et al. 2022, Front. Neurol. 12:783225) at the end of figure captions of Figs. 3.9 and 3.10

Chapter 4 in: Y. Li (ed.), Cochlear Implantation for Common Cavity Deformity, https://doi.org/10.1007/978-981-16-8217-9_4

Reference citation in line 2 of page 39 was published with incorrect caption.
Please insert Bloom et al. 2009 after Intraoperative image showing the presence of electrode array inside the IAC in a case of CC (a).

Reference citation in line 13 of page 39 was published with incorrect caption. This has now been corrected to [4.3] from [4.5].

Reference citation in line 7 of page 44 was published with incorrect caption. This has now been corrected to [above] from [below].

Chapter 5 in: Y. Li (ed.), Cochlear Implantation for Common Cavity Deformity, https://doi.org/10.1007/978-981-16-8217-9_5

Reference citation in line 17 of page 64 was published with incorrect caption. This has now been corrected to [5.16 b,c] from [5.17 b,c].

Reference citation in line 2 of page 65 was published with incorrect caption. This has now been corrected to [5.16 d-g] from [5.17 d-g].

Reference citation in line 1 of page 67 was published with incorrect caption. This has now been corrected to [5.16 h] from [5.17 h].

Chapter 7 in: Y. Li (ed.), Cochlear Implantation for Common Cavity Deformity, https://doi.org/10.1007/978-981-16-8217-9_7

Reference citation of Figs. 7.4, 7.5, 7.6, 7.7 of page 85, 86, 87, 88 was published with incorrect caption.
Please add "(reproduced with permission from Wei et al. 2022, Front. Neurol. 12:783225) at the end of figure captions of Figs. 7.4, 7.5, 7.6, 7.7.

Chapter 9 in: Y. Li (ed.), Cochlear Implantation for Common Cavity Deformity, https://doi.org/10.1007/978-981-16-8217-9_9

The affiliation of "Xinxing Fu" and "Ying Kong" should be "2, 3", and affiliation of "Yongxin Li" should be "1, 2", just like that in Chapter 10.

Printed in the United States
by Baker & Taylor Publisher Services